THE MOTHER OF ALL FIGHTS

Everything Cancer Taught Me
About Living a Full and Vibrant Life

ERIN SOTO

PURA VIDA PRESS

Copyright © 2022 by Erin Soto

All Rights Reserved, including the right to reproduce this book or portions thereof in any form whatsoever. The events are portrayed to the best of the author's memories. While all the content in this book is accurate and correct, some names and identifying characteristics of certain individuals discussed in this book have been changed to protect their privacy.

The author and the publisher do not warrant that the information in this book is fully complete and shall not be responsible for any errors or omissions.

The author and publisher shall have neither liability nor responsibility to any person or entity concerning any loss or damage caused or alleged to be caused directly or indirectly by this book.

The publisher and the author are providing this book and its contents on an "as is" basis and make no representations or warranties of any kind with respect to this book or its contents. The publisher and the author disclaim all such representations and warranties, including but not limited to warranties of healthcare for a particular purpose. In addition, the publisher and the author assume no responsibility for errors, inaccuracies, omissions, or any other inconsistencies herein.

The content of this book is for informational purposes only and is not intended to diagnose, treat, cure, or prevent any condition or disease. You understand that this book is not intended as a substitute for consultation with a licensed practitioner. Please consult with your physician or healthcare specialist regarding the suggestions and recommendations made in this book. The use of this book implies your acceptance of this disclaimer.

The publisher and the author make no guarantees concerning the level of success you may experience by following the advice and strategies contained in this book. You accept the risk that results will differ for each individual. The testimonials and examples provided in this book show exceptional results, which may not apply to the average reader. They are not intended to represent or guarantee that you will achieve the same or similar results.

Although the publisher and the author have made every effort to ensure that the information in this book was correct at press time and while this publication is designed to provide accurate information regarding the subject matter covered, the publisher and the author assume no responsibility for errors, inaccuracies, omissions, or any other inconsistencies herein and hereby disclaim any liability to any party for any loss, damage, or disruption caused by errors or omissions, whether such errors or omissions result from negligence, accident, or any other cause.

This publication is meant to be a source of valuable information for the reader; however, it is not a substitute for direct expert assistance. If such a level of assistance is required, the services of a competent professional should be sought.

First Pura Vida Press edition December 2021

Interior design by Vanessa Mendozzi

Library of Congress Cataloging-in-Publication Data has been applied for.

ISBN 979-8-9854074-0-2 (Hardback) | ISBN 979-8-9854074-1-9 (Paperback)
ISBN 979-8-9854074-2-6 (eBook) | ISBN 979-8-9854074-3-3 (Audiobook)

DEDICATION

To all those whose lives have been touched by cancer.

This book honors the taken, admires the survivors,
and supports the fighters.

It celebrates living wholeheartedly
and never giving up hope.

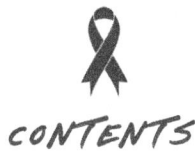

CONTENTS

INTRODUCTION	VII

PART I. WHEN THE STUDENT IS READY, THE TEACHER ARRIVES — 1
- LESSON 1. Your Body Is Trying to Tell You Something. Listen — 3
- LESSON 2. Let Yourself Be Guided — 17
- LESSON 3. Allow Yourself to Process the News — 35

PART II. HOW TO HEAL THE MIND — 53
- LESSON 4. Cancer Is a Symptom, Find the Source — 55
- LESSON 5. Mindset Is Your Greatest Medicine — 67
- LESSON 6. You Can Choose to Be Happy — 79
- LESSON 7. Release the Pressure Where You Can — 87

PART III. HOW TO HEAL THE BODY — 103
- LESSON 8. Know What You're Walking Into — 105
- LESSON 9. Find A Way to Keep Going — 123
- LESSON 10. Think About What You Put in Your Body — 137
- LESSON 11. Think About What You Put on Your Body — 151

PART IV. HOW TO HEAL THE SOUL — 157
- LESSON 12. Know When to Let Go — 159
- LESSON 13. Get in Touch with Your Soul — 173
- LESSON 14. Surround Yourself with Love — 181

PART V. THE STUDENT BECOMES THE TEACHER — 201

LESSON 15. Become a Master in Handling Setbacks — 203
LESSON 16. You Are Stronger Than You Think — 211
LESSON 17. Believe in Your Ability to Thrive — 227

EPILOGUE — 245
ABOUT THE AUTHOR — 251
ACKNOWLEDGMENTS — 253
NOTES — 257
BOOKS — 259
WEBSITES — 260

INTRODUCTION

The last thing I expected to receive in my 37th year was a Stage 3 cancer diagnosis. I had been living the average life of a busy, overly committed mom and wife when the illness began to ravage my body, steal my identity, and damage almost everything that I held dear.

If you'd asked me just two short years ago what made my life meaningful, I would have said, "Easy! My husband, our children, friends, and family."

But then along came cancer and threatened all those things. I was suddenly facing my life being cruelly interrupted and seeming to spiral out of control. I knew that my life might be cut short, so I needed to find a way to live beyond my cancer.

After wrangling with tremendous grief, fear, and heartbreak, I determined that the best way to find meaning would be through embracing whatever life I had left. This would require traveling to new depths within myself.

Of course, my family was my greatest reason for living and, while cancer sucks, I also believed in my strength and capabilities. And so, I made a promise to them and to myself that I was going to do everything in my power to survive.

I was going to use this experience as an opportunity to get deeply present with my life, connect with my body, and engage with the world. Even if I died, I would have lived a truly meaningful life as the greatest version of myself, leaving a proud legacy for my family, especially my children.

More importantly, I realized that I could do all of this despite the chaos surrounding me.

That is why I'm here writing to you today. Because I know I'm not the only one who has faced a life crisis. I also know that I'm not the only one whose life has lost meaning along the way.

During my time in the hospital, I made a promise that was I to somehow make it through this health catastrophe, I would one day tell my story and show how the most ordinary of people are capable of overcoming extraordinary hardship. I would write a book that others could use as a roadmap through the journey.

And so, dear reader, I want you to know that you are not alone in the messy work of seeking meaning in your life, and I want you to live yours wildly free and on purpose. This book is meant to help you listen to your inner voice as it says: "Today is the day to start living like you mean it."

So here you are at the starting line. You are about to build the solid foundation for what may be your greatest struggle. This is where you will turn your worst experiences into opportunities for growth. Within these pages you'll learn how to use the power of the human spirit to develop the mindset needed to overcome catastrophe.

There's an unequivocal lesson for living that I try to encourage others to learn. My ultimate goal is to make you, the reader, want to jump out of your chair and feel more alive today than ever before. I want you to redefine previously held beliefs and concepts about how best to live wholeheartedly.

If you only get one chance to live in this big, beautiful world, wouldn't you want to spend time exploring how to get more out of your life? Embracing it? Challenging it? Learning from it? Yep, me too.

There's such an enchantment about following your dreams. There is a kind of magic in the mystery of not knowing what's coming next. That's the kind of adventure that I now live for. I hardly know what I'll be doing tomorrow because I live for today — the only thing we're all promised. I am embracing every nook and cranny of life: the good, the bad, the happy, and the sad. I have never felt more alive than I do today.

Remember that year when your number one goal was to survive?

Oh yeah, that's right now! Don't they often say that what doesn't kill you makes you stronger? I'm betting on stronger.

So, here's to making new memories, crossing off unfulfilled wishes, taking calculated risks, brushing aside uncertainty for the future, and skipping down the path less traveled to expand your horizons while daring to discover just how beautiful this thing called life really is.

What you'll come to notice, if you haven't already, is that cancer is a great teacher. When facing down our fragility, cancer teaches us so many lessons about what it means to live.

I want to share with you the lessons it has taught me so that you can notice the ones it's trying to teach you. Some may match mine, some may differ, but we can take this journey together. We can learn together. We can create our best selves together.

Each chapter of your life is a lesson. Here are mine.

PART I

When the Student is Ready,
the Teacher Arrives

LESSON 1

YOUR BODY IS TRYING TO TELL YOU SOMETHING. LISTEN

I have always been a light sleeper, but the wine from Thanksgiving's evening dinner caught me off-guard, and I slept more deeply than my usual slumber. Little did I know that my comfort wouldn't last for long.

"Ouch! What's that?" Something disturbed my peace, and I was sure the cry for help was coming from inside my body.

I woke up, still dizzy from the wine, and I was disoriented. Before this, I'd never felt my heart pounding this crazily. It was as if it was demanding to get out of my body or explode in place.

I couldn't put two and two together, but then there it was. That shooting pain somewhere in my stomach, followed by blurred vision. My head was spinning.

"What was in that wine?" I thought to myself. The intensity of pain was growing with every second, sending chills down my spine.

It hurt so bad that I had to place both of my hands on top of my stomach, just below my rib cage. I tried to calm my body down by applying some pressure over that area.

"Could it be food poisoning?" The thought crossed my mind as I tried to fight back with all the strength I had. I was sure I hadn't eaten anything I was allergic to.

My hands were constantly moving over my stomach to stop the pain until I felt something unusual. I opened my eyes and tried to analyze that strange sensation.

I winced when my hand moved over a hard round object. It was about an inch in diameter, protruding from just beneath the surface of my skin.

I pressed my fingers into it. It felt like I had swallowed a ping pong ball.

I was still confused when severe contractions began. It was like the pain that you experience during labor. "Am I pregnant?" NO! I knew this wasn't possible. The ache was sharp and lingering. It felt like something was stabbing with a knife over and over again, waiting for me to give up the urge to fight.

Something was just not right about this situation.

I once read a story about a lady who went into labor without ever realizing she was pregnant. She discovered this only after she had an inexplicable need to push following severe stomach pain. She was sitting on the toilet when BAM... out popped a baby!

Nope. I was confident that I was not popping out a baby, nor was I going into labor. I've had four kids and am certain I would know if I was pregnant. However, the sheer agony I was experiencing was equivalent to labor pain.

I couldn't help but wonder if maybe this is what it feels like after your appendix has burst. That's a frightening thought, but this angle seemed a little more believable than the scenario of unexpected childbirth. I decided I was going to run with it as a form of self-diagnosis.

I took deep breaths, trying to soothe away the torment while thinking that my appendix might have burst, or if it had not already, it would in just a matter of minutes. I was breathing heavily. I didn't know why, but something inside my body told me to run for my life before this shooting pain became the reason for my unfortunate death.

Sweat dripped from my temples as I clenched my fists, lips pursed. I didn't realize I was crying until tears pooled onto my pillow, wetting my cheeks.

I curled into a fetal position, lying on the far-right corner of my bed. My body was shivering from the severity of the pain.

I needed help.

"Will, wake up." Thankfully, the words escaped my lips.

Across from me, by the dim glow of the streetlamp outside our bedroom window, I could see my husband starting to move. He grumbled, half alert, clearly unamused to be getting stirred awake from his sleep.

"What?" he said. "It's the middle of the night." Irritation dripped from his deep voice.

"I know, but I'm hurting. Badly," I said. "It's my stomach. I think we might need to go to the emergency room."

"It's Thanksgiving," he said. "You probably just ate too much. Just try to go back to sleep."

Will's words only further aggravated my pain, but this wasn't an ideal situation in which to start an argument. I fought the urge to debate what was happening to me and gave a rather emphatic response.

"No, it's not something I ate," I said. "This is different."

"What about the kids?" he said. "Do you seriously want to wake all of them up right now?"

I could tell by his tone this was not an idea he was willing to entertain. He was right. How was that going to work? I envisioned waking up each of our four kids, one by one, carrying them while asleep down into the car, and then rushing Mommy to the hospital.

After giving a little more thought to how this scene might play out, it no longer seemed to me an idea worth considering, either. Everyone, but for me, was enjoying the sedative effects from the tryptophan following our turkey dinner. I didn't want to bother them. Cranky kids and a midnight adventure to the emergency room? No thanks. I've always said, "Pick your battles," and this one didn't seem worth fighting.

I resigned to accepting suffering in silence throughout the night.

As I lay in misery, my mind started swirling over the infinite possibilities of everything that could go wrong during the current state of emergency. If something inside of me had indeed ruptured, I very well might die here tonight, alone with my thoughts.

I had never thought about death. It wasn't something I'd given my attention to until now.

"Am I going to die? Is this what it feels like to fade away from everyone's lives?" I shook my head, trying to stop these thoughts from messing with my mind.

I knew that if these were my final moments, Will would be one guilty husband when he awoke and found me gone for good. My dramatics were not fostering the empathy I had hoped to receive from my better half. Nevertheless, something about the cruel idea of his guilt come morning strangely comforted me.

"If it doesn't go away by morning, we will take the kids to my parents' house and go straight to an emergency room. That's only 5 hours away. I can manage this until that time." I repeated the sentence over and over again, trying to convince myself that it sounded believable.

Every inch of my body knew that I was trying to fool it, to calm it down so I could get some sleep without waking up Will again or crying out loud. I did what the doctor told me to do during labor by practicing Lamaze. Lamaze is a breathing technique based on the idea that controlled breathing can enhance relaxation and decrease pain perception. I started focusing on taking deep breaths. I inhaled through my nose for several seconds before slowly exhaling from my mouth.

•••

"Erin, are you up? How are you feeling?" Will asked.

I slowly opened my eyes to notice the sun was now shining softly through the window. I could hear birds chirping from the trees in our backyard and realized I had survived the night.

"Seriously? Now you ask? Your timing seems rather convenient," I snapped.

I remembered the fiasco I'd suffered a few hours ago; I quickly grabbed my stomach. The ping pong ball was now gone. It had disappeared. I must have digested the mystery mass somehow during my sleep. I inspected my belly and moved my hands across my stomach to see if it had moved to somewhere else.

"Strange," I thought to myself. I had been certain we were going to be racing to the ER first thing this morning. I was rather impressed by my body's ability to naturally recover from the entire episode and was equally relieved we didn't have to waste the morning with an inconvenient trip to the hospital.

"All good. No need to panic," I said. "Your drama queen is going to be A-okay. You were right. It probably was just something I ate. Speaking of which, I'd better go for a run. Maybe this all happened because I ate too much." I smiled.

I hopped out of bed, strapped on my jogging shoes, and bounced down the stairs and out the front door. Time to burn off the copious amounts of the comfort food I had blissfully indulged in the day before. As I made my way down the sidewalk, I began thinking about what had transpired in the middle of the night before.

I considered it one of the other tummy troubles that had made me visit my doctor just the week prior. Maybe this was somehow related to the digestive problems? I should probably mention this to my doctor. Whatever that ache was last night, it was out of the ordinary and something I never wanted to experience ever again. But no matter what it was, I congratulated myself for cheating death out of one more day.

After wrapping my morning run, I sent my doctor an email detailing the whole bizarre ping pong ball incident. I'd been having digestive problems for some time now and had started to seek medical help. It all began after we returned from our summer vacation in Costa Rica back in late August. I distinctly remember the timing because I experienced my first attack on the 15-minute drive home after the first day of school drop-off. I will never forget the sheer distress I felt while sitting in never-ending traffic at the intersection a short mile from our home. Let's just say things escalated way too close to call, leaving me with an understanding of why some people depend on diapers in place of their normal underwear. Every red light on that morning's drive became a personal nemesis.

Following that adventurous episode, I started running to the toilet during all hours of the day and night. My considerate family expressed their sincere concern by making me the brunt of a slew of potty jokes. We had a great many laughs at my expense for several weeks.

"When you're sliding into first, and your pants are about to burst... diarrhea, diarrhea."

My kids would taunt me each and every time I made a mad dash for the bathroom, praying to reach the porcelain throne in time.

"Dad, she's doing it again," they would say.

My mom and husband had started pointing out the increasing amount of time I spent using the bathroom. It was starting to become an inconvenience and was not as funny as we all had once thought.

These attacks were now happening as often as five to six times a day. No place was safe from their wrath. I quickly memorized every restroom along the path of our usual family stops: the grocery store, kids' school, football stadium, soccer and softball fields. Every last one of these had become fair game to rush to whenever the 'urge to splurge' came crashing in.

This went on for months. I knew I should probably see a doctor, but what was I going to say? The thought of calling to request an appointment for diarrhea was humiliating enough to deter me from ever doing so.

I would imagine the conversation and shudder in horror. "Hi, it's Erin Soto. I need to schedule an appointment. What for? I've been suffering from chronic diarrhea for several months."

I knew nothing is funny when it involves the doctors and hospitals. Still, the jokes my family had been cracking over my diarrhea problem were enough to give me nightmares about how it might sound even to the health professionals.

I could hear them laughing whenever I thought about making an appointment. Each time I'd decide to pass, telling myself I was way too busy to call. I could always do it tomorrow, next week, or wait another month. I'd tell myself I would eventually get the nerve to schedule an appointment if the problem failed to clear up independently.

"Anyway, it's not like this is an emergency. People have diarrhea all the time." Maybe not for as long or often as I had been experiencing, but what was the worst-case scenario we could be facing here? Nothing I was overly concerned with.

I was certain this would boil down to something like needing to make a simple change in diet. Maybe I had developed a food allergy or gluten intolerance. "That makes perfect sense. Gluten is the latest devil, according to the hype diet advice everyone is following nowadays. So, I'll try eating less of it. Cut back on the cheese. Easy peasy. That ought to make for a quick fix and solution to my problems."

Besides, I was slammed juggling our family's schedule. Fall is always our busiest season. There was not a single line open on our over-scheduled calendar to fit in one more commitment.

Our four kids are involved in anywhere from three to five extracurricular activities at any given time. Their schedules always took precedence. We had paid good money for them to participate in these activities, and I intended to get full value or at least make the most out of it.

Between their health checkups, orthodontist trips, dental appointments, parent-teacher conferences, birthday parties, music lessons, and way more many sports than I could recount, there simply was not enough time to tackle my never-ending to-do list.

I'm sure that even Mary Poppins herself would have considered our calendar highly offensive. I was drowning in overwhelm and failing miserably at following through on our family commitments.

"The doctor's visit can wait," I kept telling myself. I could hold it off until Thanksgiving break, when everything slowed down enough to come up for some air. That was the end of fall sports, when my focus transferred over to holiday duties. The fall holiday break provided a minor reprieve from the hustle, offering just enough time to allow me to finally schedule myself an appointment, should this issue still pose a problem. As it would turn out, this was still a problem come November.

I was no stranger to chaos and was swamped. I often fantasize about the lost freedom of the spare time I used to have when I worked at my former full-time job. Back when I could sneak off for a cup of coffee with a co-worker, listen to an entire audible book, or blast 90s hip hop during my long commute to and from the office. And sneak in errands over my lunch break without any kids in tow. I'd spent almost eight years working for The Walt Disney Company in various business development and marketing roles on the Burbank studio lot.

I was eventually promoted to full-time mom-ager for our family of six after our youngest, Liam, was born. It was a lot less glamorous a gig than my former professional career working for an entertainment mogul. Still, I had worked my way up to the most difficult job there is in life. Raising my four minions full-time turned out to be quite the increase in workload, but there was a sign-on bonus in savings for no longer paying the high-cost of childcare.

My stay-at-home mom transition was the best decision for our family. The lack of having an actual parent at home to cook, launder, clean, help with homework, and cart the kids around to their many activities had become a serious point of contention. Calculating how much of my income we were left with after the expense of gas, commute time, and our beloved nanny's salary ultimately led us to decide to transition to the DIY route.

I had anticipated how wonderful it would be after I could finally stay home and care for my family. Years of 'working mom guilt' were something I knew all too well. I can't tell you how many times my kids would complain that I never had the time to join them on their class field trips or to assist as a volunteer at Friday Art Center "like all the other kids' moms." I remember feeling envious of those ladies in their yoga pants and tennis attire during morning drop-offs in the school parking lot. They always looked so well put together and relaxed.

Meanwhile, I'd be rushing my kids through the car line, stressing about getting onto the Interstate to begin my two-hour commute from South Orange County. It was not uncommon for me to have fruit loops stuck in my hair and a coffee-stained work shirt by 7 am. When I looked down at my messy self while pulling into work, I would often discover my pants were on inside out, or that I accidentally was wearing two left shoes.

Those other moms had it so easy. They never seemed to hold a care in the world or have the need to rush off to someplace they were required to be. I imagined they all went to brunch for hours after the school parking lot emptied. What I would have given to join them and skip out on my usual daily grind in rush hour.

I daydreamed about how productive I would be should I ever get to stay at home. I had so many big plans in store for what I would do with all that magical spare time. Our house would be immaculate. Errands would be run while kids were at school, without them weighing down my shopping cart, throwing tantrums in the aisles, or asking to use the bathroom yet again. No, I would slowly peruse the aisles of Target without high blood pressure pulsing through my veins from kids asking if we could buy every bright and shiny object that caught their attention as we passed. It would be glorious.

Of course, I was in for a brutal reality check after the stay-at-home transition finally occurred. I quickly discovered that my new job came without lunch breaks and lacked adult conversation, connection, and stimulus. I was lucky if I left the house with my hair and teeth brushed. This was especially true during the season when I had a baby on one hip and a preschooler on the other, always present and needing my constant attention.

For years I had missed out on milestone firsts for the kids, seeing those through texts sent by my nanny while I worked away at the office. I used to envy her experiencing everything, but I now had the honor of being present myself. I, of course, appreciated the difficult challenge I now faced for the many privileges it offered. And I also realized we hadn't paid our nanny nearly enough. This whole stay-at-home-mom gig was so much harder than I had envisioned.

A far cry from the fantasy I had created in my head. Zero pay and very little recognition or thanks for all the hard work. The grass is always greener, so they say.

That said, I truly valued my special time with my youngest, Liam, when the other kids were at school. I had missed so many precious moments for my other three, such as witnessing their first steps and first words. Those had happened with the other kids while I was working. This full-time mom role for four was tough, but so worthwhile. After several years I seemed to be getting a better handle on balancing my responsibilities, and I did a rather decent job juggling my many tasks.

The stay-at-home chaos was one of the reasons why I didn't prioritize the time to seek medical advice from my doctor or place self-care above my family's needs. This brings us back to my waiting far too long to finally schedule my long overdue doctor's appointment.

I was in denial, and I made up many excuses. It was a combination of both. The truth is, I just wasn't concerned that the symptoms I had been experiencing were red flags warranting medical attention. They were easy enough to dismiss and nothing I considered to be significant.

・・・

I had managed to put off seeing my doctor for more than four months. That worked until the changes in bowel movements escalated to severe constipation. The bloating discomfort that accompanied this was worse than the inconvenience of chronic diarrhea.

I was also growing tired of hearing my mom and husband complain about how much precious time I had been wasting the last few months while sitting on the toilet. It was starting to become a trigger of frustration for everyone in the family. That was what ultimately led me to finally decide to go in and have myself checked out.

After constantly delaying my appointment with a doctor because I was too embarrassed to check in at a hospital to ask for treatment for diarrhea, finally I had landed an appointment with our family care practitioner, Dr. Travis. I sat on the exam table, recounting all the humiliating stories and symptoms I had been experiencing.

I decided it was finally time to face what I had been running from. It had become a do-or-die thing for me. I couldn't keep up with the potty jokes anymore. Will and my mom seemed increasingly worried over the continued inconvenience and discomfort I was going through.

For full transparency, I admit that I wasn't playing the role of a helpful patient with my doctor. In my discomfort over explaining issues concerning my bowel movements, I glazed over the list of many symptoms. I resorted to providing him with a brief summation of why I was seeking medical advice by sharing our family's favorite potty jokes and trying to laugh off the embarrassment. It was easier to laugh than to discuss the awkward details of my digestive system.

I recall wanting to get the heck out of the office as soon as I had arrived. I hated visiting the doctor under usual circumstances. Bowel problems being the purpose of this visit only made it all that much worse to endure. I wanted to get through this appointment quickly and right back to my daily hustle as fast as possible. So, first, check it off the list to appease my family's concerns, proving I had indeed been seen by my doctor as advised. Then, ideally, share that all is well and move along on my merry way.

"I was reviewing the documents from your annual physical assessment from last June and everything appears to be in working order," Dr. Travis said. "I did notice something a little off on your lab work. You are anemic. Are you still struggling with feeling tired and sluggish? Have the folate supplements I suggested you try out helped with this?"

"Funny you should ask. I tried taking the extra iron pills that you suggested. They haven't helped much with my low energy, though," I said.

"Then again," I thought to myself, "no magic pill can fix the fact that I have four kids." Keeping them alive and well is an ever exhausting and daunting effort. No wonder I'm always so tired. Not surprising. I had been a walking zombie for the last eleven years, ever since I entered motherhood.

Of course, it wasn't the kids' fault that they needed their mother to feed and care for them. And it was something I loved and enjoyed doing.

I regularly complained to Will that the extreme fatigue from the sleepless nights of caring for a newborn never seemed to fade with time after we had Liam. He was now four years old, and even though he had been sleeping through the night for years, my exhaustion level only seemed to be getting worse.

I got out of bed every morning feeling completely drained and ready to collapse, seemingly the same level of exhaustion I'd felt when crawling into bed the night before after a long day. Waking up tired and drained of energy was now becoming routine. I didn't know why things were going wrong. I was a mess without knowing how to fix myself.

I had accepted extreme fatigue as my new normal. I figured this is what people mean when they talk about feeling tired with age. Of course, I never expected it to be this bad in my mid-30s; but someday, maybe when the kids grew a little older and more independent, I would wake up to discover that my former zest had miraculously returned. A girl can always dream.

"You mentioned you had just been on vacation in Costa Rica over the summer, is that right?" Dr. Travis asked. "Right before all of your symptoms began."

"Yes," I said. "Why? Could there be some kind of a connection?"

"Based on the symptoms you have described, there is a possibility your stomach troubles could be from parasites," he said. "It happens more often than you might think. People return from traveling to tropical places and have been known to bring back unwelcome stowaways in the form of parasites. They attack your system in various ways. You likely wouldn't have ever realized this had happened to you. It could have been while swimming in shallow infested waters, like a river or mangrove."

That jogged my memory. I thought of doing exactly that at the beach in Playa Cabrillo. I sat in the shallow water at the edge, where the river flowed into the ocean, and splashed around for hours with the kids, safely away from the waves and rip current. I considered it Mother Nature's toddler pool. I distinctly recalled noticing all sorts of little bugs floating around in the foam on top of the water and thinking how it seemed full of questionable insects. A cesspool for tiny parasites looking to invade and prey on unsuspecting tourists. Great! I had done this all to myself.

Parasites! Gross. This may be worse than I thought.

I've seen the television program Monsters Inside Me. It's one of my kids' favorite shows to watch. Just before our family trip, we happened to catch a particularly traumatic episode. This lady had traveled to Costa Rica for her bachelorette party. While hiking, they presume, a bot fly landed on the back of her neck and laid its eggs just beneath her skin, all while going undetected.

Several weeks later, on the day of her wedding, no less, all the larvae began to hatch, and she could hear and feel bot fly babies crawling around inside of her head. True story!

The stuff of nightmares, right? You'd better believe I'd slathered our bodies with copious amounts of bug spray during our trip, fully intent on deterring bot flies. But, unfortunately, parasites attacking from inside water were not something that had occurred to me — nasty little buggers.

"Don't worry. It's a quick fix." Dr. Travis said. "We simply have to identify what kind of parasite you have. We'll test you for all of them. Then it is as easy as prescribing strong medication to eradicate them. We can quickly resolve the problem. First, though, you have to collect a stool sample for the lab, so we know what we are dealing with here."

"Lovely," I said. "I can hardly wait."

I almost laughed as I responded. The trip to the doctor was a success. Nothing like I had expected, but telling the kids that their mom had monsters inside was going to be a huge hit, given their fondness for the show. And thinking that Mommy had such monsters inside would divert their attention away from my frequent restroom trips. A welcome change of topic from the onslaught of toilet jokes I had grown accustomed to. We were running out of fresh potty humor material.

I picked up my prescription from the pharmacy on my way home. While collecting a fecal sample for what I believed to be a case of parasitic poop, I realized something could be wrong. There was a slight tinge of blood in my stool. The stool was noticeably dark black as I examined it through the test tube. Admiring excrement matter was not a habit of mine. I tended to wipe and flush without paying close attention. This was the first time I recognized that my bowel movements appeared abnormal.

I knew that finding blood in your stool was usually a bad sign. I considered this more fascinating than problematic at the time. These parasites must be more mischievous than anticipated.

"I'd better get the sample back to the lab to get whatever potent pack of pills is needed to wipe away the unwelcome visitors. I refuse to serve as their host for another day." I thought about them reproducing, multiplying, and invading my insides. It was time to evict the pests for overstaying their welcome.

The day just before Thanksgiving, I received an email from my doctor. He said that my lab results were ready for review. I quickly opened the email to learn what kind of monsters we were dealing with, only to find that they had tested for pages of possible parasites and every single one had tested as negative.

Now that parasites were ruled out, I emailed my doctor regarding the painful ping pong to see if we could follow up with another visit and continue investigating this matter. It seemed to be escalating.

He replied to my message explaining he had placed an order for a procedure called a flexible sigmoidoscopy. It was a less intrusive form of a colonoscopy and was being ordered to rule out digestive problems. He explained that we would determine in what direction it was best to go after receiving the results.

From that moment onward, I knew there was something wrong with my body. After seeing the blood in my stool sample, I was almost sure the diarrhea problem was not normal. I needed to get myself fixed.

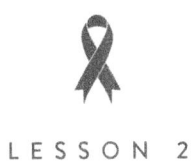

LESSON 2

LET YOURSELF BE GUIDED

When Dr. Travis mentioned sigmoidoscopy, I was left to figure out what could be so wrong that I had to go through such an elaborate ordeal. It wasn't that I was having issues so much with the procedure itself, but never in the slightest figment of my imagination had it occurred to me that I would be going for such a procedure in my late-30s. In contrast, I have seen elders going through this procedure. My dad used to joke it was a rite of passage into your golden years. Although the process was not that complicated, what irked me was the preparatory work required to exhume every food particle resting in there, either digested or undigested.

Digestive problems seemed far less disturbing than parasites. I dialed the number from the email to schedule an appointment. It was early on a Monday morning, and I had just returned home after dropping the kids off at school. The health center explained to me that they had just coincidentally received a cancellation for the very next day.

They advised me to take it; otherwise, it would be about four to six weeks until their next available opening. The nurse told me that if I agreed to take the available slot, I would have to begin the preparatory process for the flexible sigmoidoscopy immediately. Still, there was time enough considering I had not yet eaten. We had a full 24 hours until the procedure. I took the appointment.

The nurse explained that I needed to carefully review an email she was about to send that detailed everything I would need to complete before the next morning. I wasn't permitted to eat any solid food and would need to adhere to a strict clear liquid diet. The thought of bailing out on the lasagna that I was now preparing for dinner later that night made my stomach rumble, as the delicious aroma in the kitchen was only spiking my appetite.

I drove to the pharmacy to pick up my prescription for a medication I would need to drink later that afternoon. The nurse had instructed me to follow the directions very closely; I might have to repeat the entire procedure if I failed to prepare properly. I had no clue what I was in for and happily agreed.

The next 24 hours were a blur of hunger and bathroom dashes, the latter causing even more embarrassment than the preceding months of potty jokes combined. It was not pretty, but I'll spare you the worst of it.

The next morning, I felt weak and emaciated from the starvation of the liquid diet that I had now been on for 24 hours. The restroom trips left me with no energy to stand. I stood in the shower with water washing over me, leaning against the wall to avoid fainting.

My stomach was still rumbling as I daydreamed about all I wanted to eat for dinner later that night. We were going to celebrate my surviving this hideous incident over a spread of solid food. "What shall it be?" The tantalizing possibilities of delicious ideas had me eager with anticipation. My kids were busy dressing themselves, completing their school morning grind, when I yelled from the shower, announcing "Tonight, we shall feast!"

No doubt, I was delirious, crazed, and still a bit confused from all that had occurred, so I thought it would be best to allow my husband to tackle most of the parental duties that morning. Unfortunately, the mere process of getting myself ready and dressed took what remaining energy and focus I still had. I tried to ignore the pounding headache I was now suffering due to hunger. I wasn't allowed even a tiny sip of water that morning because of the anesthesia.

Thankfully, my pre-op required that we check in early, at 8 am. We all moved quickly through the morning routine to make it out the door on time to drop off the kids along the way to my appointment.

We made it to the hospital just in time to check in, and Will was allowed to accompany me as my plus one. A sigmoidoscopy requires someone to drive you home for safety as this involves twilight anesthesia with a mild dose of sedation.

...

I had never been behind the doors of the Gastroenterology Center before. All I knew were the stories my dad had shared with me after his first procedure post-retirement. In my mind, this was usually done on older men and not young ladies.

Upon seeing the sheer number of patients awaiting their turn, I realized that this center was run like a well-oiled machine. The hospital I was in processed fifty or more appointments each day, and I was yet another in a long assembly line of clients. No wonder there was a six-week wait just to land the next reservation. This place was snowballing. Everyone was moving in and out, running around with extreme efficiency to allow as many people as possible to receive their screenings in a timely fashion.

I was grateful to have Will there with me. He was even permitted to join me in the preparation area rather than remain outside in the waiting room. I appreciated having him there for moral support. I started to feel a little nervous as reality settled in while they checked my vitals and began to admit me as a patient.

As instructed by my nurse, I undressed, put on a hospital gown with the flap open in the back, and proceeded to model it around behind the privacy curtain while asking Will for his honest opinion as to whether he thought the yellow hospital socks clashed with the bluish hue of my gown.

"Do you think this opening in the back might be a little too revealing?" I asked. "Be honest, if you catch my drift."

I smiled at him while trying to break the ice of the serious nature of our scenario. Before he could answer, a nurse interrupted our conversation, entered my personal medical information into the system, and then inserted my intravenous line.

The curtain again swished open, and in walked a fresh-faced gastroenterologist in her early 30s. Her hair was shiny and pulled nicely back into a ponytail. I noticed that her complexion was glowing. She had large brown eyes, tan skin, a very pretty face, and she carried herself with a kind and comforting demeanor. I could see an adorable baby bump protruding from under her scrubs, popping out ever so slightly between the openings of her white lab coat. I assumed she must be around her third trimester. Seeing her reminded me of the days when I used to be a working mom.

"Hello, I'm Dr. Dalal," she said. "You must be Erin. I will be performing today's procedure. I have read Dr. Travis's report, and it sounds like we are here to rule out some digestive problems for you."

I gave her the short version of my symptoms, and she explained how the flexible sigmoidoscopy would work. She would be using a narrow tube with a tiny camera on one end to look inside my lower colon.

"Just to clarify," I said. "I will be fast asleep throughout this, right?"

"Correct," she said. "It's quite common for us to diagnose something like diverticulitis or other digestive problems during this process. So, we may have an answer for you just as soon as you wake up. The entire procedure should only take about 20 minutes."

"Excellent news," I said.

"If you don't have any other questions, the procedure room is just about ready for you, so I'm going to finish up on some final preparations. I'll see you in there shortly."

My husband was preoccupied with working on his phone, answering emails and texts from clients. Both of us were eager to breeze through this appointment so we could get back to business as usual. Nevertheless, he paused just in time to quickly kiss me goodbye on the cheek and wished me luck as the nurse wheeled me away down the hall.

As soon as the doors to the procedure room opened, I could feel butterflies in my stomach. Then the nerves settled in, and I was feeling apprehensive. The scene in front of me reminded me a lot of when I had gone in for my cesarean section years ago when my twins were born. The room was cold and had bright light fixtures hanging on the ceiling, hovering above an operating table. The medical team of two attending nurses, Dr. Dalal and my anesthesiologist, were busily preparing for my arrival.

The nurse took a moment to introduce herself and the others and then instructed me to lay down on the table and remain on my left side during this procedure. She told me I should make myself as comfortable as possible. She explained how this required curling my legs up into my stomach with my bare bum facing out for all to see and access.

"Whoa there, Cowpokes. Hold your horses," I said. "Shouldn't we at least get to know each other a little better here first? Call me old-fashioned, but I know exactly where you all plan on venturing to in the coming minutes, and I feel inclined to let you know that I like long walks on the beach at sunset and enjoy Thai food."

"Very cute," she said. "Now, let's help you onto the table."

After having birthed four children into the world, this wasn't my first rodeo requiring me to expose my private she-parts. On several occasions I've been in rooms like this one, full of strangers asking me to expose my hoo-ha and hidey-hole for all to kindly see. It seems that, as you age, and if you are going through common health procedures that require a detailed examination of your reproductive or anorectal anatomy, you have no option left but to allow others to invade your privacy.

Childbirth is far worse than a sigmoidoscopy. While I felt em-bare-assed (pun intended) by their instructions, I reminded myself that they see and do this daily. This place had practically a revolving door for the procedure. I needed to swallow my pride, act obediently, and follow their command. My lady-parts were nothing they hadn't seen many times before, nor would mine likely be worth remembering. It wouldn't offer a welcome change from their usual clientele. I awkwardly climbed onto the table and assumed the position.

"Erin, can you please confirm that this is your medical record number on the screen and tell us your full name and birthdate?

"Erin Claridge Soto. June 18, 1982."

"Great! It looks like we are all in the right operating room," she said. "Lastly, can you please confirm the name of the procedure you are here for today?"

Crap. What was the medical name? It was something long that I couldn't remember under all this pressure.

"Yes," I said. "You are about to use that scope-ma-jig thing right there and violate my exit-only zone. In layman's terms, of course."

"A flexible sigmoidoscopy." Dr. Dalal said.

That was the proper name. I was sure Dr. Dalal cracked a little smile when she answered. Success! I had made her laugh.

"Okay, Erin. You seem well and ready. Time for us to get started."

The anesthesiologist next asked what my favorite cocktail was. "That's a funny question to ask," I thought to myself.

"Well, I'm more of a wine connoisseur, but for the sake of being a team player, let's go with a margarita."

"Excellent selection," he said. "I'm about to give you the best margarita you have ever had. Can you count backward from five to one for me, please?"

"I'll drink to that," I said. "Bottoms up. Five, fourrrrrr..." Darkness.

• • •

I started to stir and could hear a soft beeping noise in the background. Again, I felt hazy and discombobulated. Then, finally, I opened my eyes and could see the back of Dr. Dalal. She stood speaking to one of the nurses whose finger was touching the video screen monitor.

As my vision started coming into focus, I could make out a strange slimy white tunnel object surrounded by the blackness they were all fixated on and seemed to be talking about. Everyone was busy concentrating on what they were discussing. So much so that they seemed almost too preoccupied to notice that I was beginning to come out of the anesthesia cocktail.

Just as I was piecing the bits together of where I was and what was going on, I recall hearing the anesthesiologist say he was administering more medicine and I quickly slipped back out of consciousness.

The next time I awoke, they were ready. This time a nurse was waiting for me a few inches in front of my face.

"Hello, Erin. How are you feeling?" she said. "Looks like you are starting to wake up for us. We needed to monitor you here for a few minutes after we had to administer extra medicine. It has taken you some time to wake up from that. Sorry, you popped in on us there for a moment during your procedure. We are ready to bring you back into the other room for recovery. I'll bet your husband is wondering where we all have been."

I could feel the effects of the anesthesia; my mouth was dry, and I was slightly nauseous. But, on the bright side, I was so doped up I somehow had forgotten how hungry I was. As they wheeled me through the hallway, I glanced over to see other patients recovering behind their privacy curtains. A man with gray hair in his early 50s looked glazed over while a nurse tended to him. I wondered if I looked as out of sorts as he did.

We made our way back to my recovery space, where Will was eagerly awaiting our arrival. He seemed relieved to see us.

"That took a long time," Will said. "I thought it was only supposed to be 20 minutes. I was starting to get nervous over here."

The nurse looked at my husband and gave him an awkward smile as she positioned me and my rolling table, locking it safely into place.

"Yes. We ended up requiring a lengthier procedure than we had originally anticipated. Once Erin is a little more awake, Dr. Dalal will be coming in to speak with both of you. We want to make sure she has a little more time to finish processing the anesthesia out of her system. We would like her to be a little more coherent for post-procedure conversation. The doctor will be in to speak with you shortly."

Will proceeded to rub my hand where the IV had been and asked how I was feeling.

"I can't wait to go home."

∙ ∙ ∙

Will and I sat together quietly, waiting for a few minutes until the curtain was pulled back and Dr. Dalal entered. This time she wasn't smiling, and her demeanor seemed to have drastically changed. Instead, she had a somber expression on her face that made both Will and me glance at one another anxiously.

"Hi, Erin. I hope you are feeling better," she said. "I want to speak with you about what we found during today's procedure. I was able to check the lower part of your colon. About 6-8 inches up into your sigmoid colon, I found something concerning. It explains a lot as to why you've been having all your bowel problems. You have a mass that is about 2 inches in diameter blocking your lower colon. I was able to take several biopsies of this mass and will be sending these off to the lab immediately. It may take several days before we receive the results."

Hearing her mention a mass of 2 inches instantly reminded me of the ping pong ball that put me through so much trouble that night of sheer agony. It all made sense. I'd assumed that the ball had vanished, but it was still there. I was thankful that it hadn't resurfaced to make me go through that pain all over again.

Dr. Dalal explained how she needed to get a better look to see if she could find anything else throughout the rest of my entire colon. She asked that I come back for her to perform a full colonoscopy the next day. This second procedure would also include examining the large intestine so she could look for more inflammation, ulcers, or abnormal growths and polyps. She needed to use a colonoscope to examine further up, to see what she'd been limited in seeing during today's procedure.

She further explained that she'd ordered a CT scan to get another perspective of the mass and had also placed an order for blood work that I would need to have taken in the lab on our way out. The seriousness of her tone was making me apprehensive, and I could feel my gut going all alert and screaming BAD NEWS!!! She re-emphasized that she needed to perform a full colonoscopy to know more. The nursing staff had managed to schedule me in for this follow-up procedure first thing the very next morning.

Wait!!! So, I have to do this all over again? That means I wouldn't be able to eat again and would have to remain on the liquid diet while choking down another gallon of that nasty colon prep juice. I was picking up on her sense of urgency while being equally surprised with how they could schedule me to be seen again so quickly. I reluctantly agreed, with the sole desire of being discharged so I could go home and rest.

...

During the next morning's procedure, I did not wake up while the colonoscopy was in action. After I was wheeled back into the recovery area with Will anxiously awaiting, this time Dr. Dalal returned, seeming even more distressed than she had the day before.

"I have some positive news, which is that I did not find anything else that I hadn't already discovered during yesterday's flex sig. You had a few small polyps that I was able to remove," she said. "I also took some extra images and biopsies of the mass again, to get a second test out of extra precaution."

She went on to add that she had scheduled an appointment for me with a surgeon for this coming Monday morning.

"Wait a minute! Did she just mention surgery?" I thought to myself. She continued on, noting I had not yet completed the lab work she'd ordered the day before. She emphasized that she needed me to go in and have it all done immediately. Same with the CT scan she had ordered. This was to be done STAT, as in, right now...today.

"There aren't any openings here in Radiology at the Irvine hospital for a CT scan." She had made some calls and managed to schedule an urgent appointment for one about half an hour away at a sister hospital in Anaheim. They could see me in the next two hours and expected me to arrive within the hour to prepare. Dr. Dalal stated that we needed to go directly there. She had rushed my discharge to accommodate our need to hurry to this next appointment.

Will and I looked at each other, lost in suspense. Things sure felt to be moving rather quickly. The genuine concern and sincerity in Dr. Dalal's tone hit a lot harder than it had the day before. I had been so distraught thinking of another evening of colon prep and the need to return for a second procedure that I'd failed to recognize she meant business when she had ordered blood work and a CT scan.

We had both somehow managed to miss the sense of urgency around everything else we were supposed to have already tackled by this point. I was now feeling incredibly frail after two days of tests, procedures, and the liquid diet, as well as this second day's dose of anesthesia. I wasn't clear-headed, but the impression Dr. Dalal made was direct enough and to the point: going home right now and following through later was not an option.

She wasn't offering advice in the form of a request. This had escalated into a state of emergency. She gave me the approval to eat food, suggesting we pick up something on the way and take it along to the hospital. I stopped in the lab on the first floor for more needle pricks to collect blood, and then we were allowed to leave the hospital en route to the next stop in Anaheim. As hungry as I had been after going into my third day without food, the only thing I could fathom tolerating following the anesthesia was soup. Hence, more liquid. So, we picked up some wonton soup for the drive.

As we pulled into the medical center, we entered the parking structure directly past the first building on the right, with a sign out front that read Infusion Center. I watched as a woman helped a frail man exit the door. He seemed sickly and needed to hold onto her arm for balance.

I'd been to this hospital many times before and had never noticed the infusion center building until this day. I felt a little sorry for myself as Will helped me up and out of the car and assisted me in walking into the building, much like the frail man I'd just seen who seemed in a similar fragile state.

Will helped check me in at reception. I was asked to sit in a waiting area where someone would meet us to provide more liquid medication that I would need to consume within the next hour.

I was out of sorts, and both Will and I were too afraid to say very much to one another. Neither of us wanted to talk about the thoughts we both were thinking. We knew something was possibly very wrong but, in our home, we tend to work under the philosophy that we shouldn't hit the panic button until we have a genuine reason to stress.

Both of us have had false-positive results with biopsies in the past. We had allowed ourselves to get worked up during the waiting period for results, only to discover the results were benign. A minor procedure had been required in the worst instance; there had always been a quick fix. Wasting energy fussing over something that could turn out to be nothing worth worrying over in the first place was pointless. I was young and seemingly healthy. This was probably nothing more than a false alarm.

We agreed that we were going to treat this in the same way. Sure, a little distressing, but why allow ourselves to ponder the endless trail of what-if scenarios? We decided we weren't going to say anything to the kids. They didn't need to know all that Mommy was going through this week. It might scare them as much as it was frightening both of us. We were going to play it cool. After this CT scan, we would return home, resume usual activities, and wait until we received the results for both procedures.

We sat in the waiting room and listened to a pianist playing peaceful classical music, which served as the intended calming distraction. Will held my hand, and I rested my head on his shoulder. I was cold and faint, and he covered me with his jacket to comfort me as I drank the contents of the bottle of liquid the radiology tech had just delivered.

The tech had explained this was a special dye called contrast material needed for my CT scan. He said that soft tissues wouldn't show up without drinking this and that it was going to help the mass in my colon appear white on the scan. So, it was more like illuminating my insides, highlighting my blood vessels, organs, and other structures.

I drank the oral solution to enhance the scan, and just before the scan itself they injected a drug directly into my veins to help everything they intended to search for better stand out in the image.

They were going to light me up just like the Fourth of July.

The technician administered my third IV in the last 48 hours and brought me into another cold room where I had to lie down on another table. During the test, I was slowly pushed into a doughnut-shaped machine.

The scanner was humming loudly, and I could hear it circulating around my body. The radiology technician spoke to me through a speaker: I would be instructed to inhale a deep breath and hold it for several seconds before I could exhale. Movement can blur the image, so I was also told I needed to remain very still.

After a few minutes inside the machine, the radiographer joked that he had made sure to capture images of my good side and that this session was a wrap. He also told me I needed to drink as much water as possible to help my kidneys flush out the contrast material from my body. After that, I finally returned home to await the results.

Considering Dr. Dalal's urgency for needing this scan, I assumed that the results would be serious, and that had me anxiously awaiting them. Remaining cool, calm, and collected over the next few days became a challenge for me, as I was on my own. Will needed to immediately return to work in order to catch up after several days of caring for me. I had a tough time trying to get through my usual daily activities. I was understandably scatterbrained while waiting to receive both the biopsy and CT scan results.

It was now Thursday of that action-packed week. I attempted to remain as productive as possible and kept myself occupied by cleaning the house, running errands, and chauffeuring the kids to their after-school activities. By the time Friday morning had arrived, however, I chose to stop trying to distract myself with busy work and killing time while the kids were in school, deciding it was best for an impromptu visit with my parents for comfort and support.

• • •

My family history is twisted and funny, but I am thankful for having a rather large, supportive, and caring family. My mom and stepdad had recently moved to our neighborhood in Southern California, relocating from the San Francisco Bay area. My mom had retired, and after spending the last 35 years working, she was delighted to finally join my stepdad in the golden years of retirement life. I had somehow managed to convince them to relocate near us to be closer to their grandkids. I was still adjusting to the many perks of having my parents as neighbors. The idea was that I could now help them over this next season in their life, and we could enjoy spending quality time together regularly rather than just during short visits for holidays.

I grew up just north of the Golden Gate Bridge in Novato, a town bordering the wine country and Napa Valley. I had a mostly picture-perfect childhood there. In addition to my mom and stepdad, my family includes four siblings and my dad and stepmom, all of whom remain in Northern California.

My parents were college sweethearts and were married for 15 years before their divorce. The idea of my dad and mom ever being married is puzzling to make sense of because, if you ever met my parents, you would quickly see how they are opposites.

My dad is a laid-back tie-dyed-shirt-wearing, Birkenstock donning, pickleball playing, chilled-out dude who worked as a master control engineer at KPIX Channel 5, San Francisco's CBS affiliate, for the majority of his professional career. I joined him there one summer during college, working as an intern for the television station's Communications Director. Dad, now, is also enjoying recent retirement and grandparent privileges closer to my sister and brothers up north. When I was a little girl, he was always very hands-on and involved. He had energy for days and loved to paint my sister's and my nails, cooked, cleaned our house, helped me with homework, and volunteered with Girl Scouts. He tried to be present at all of his kids' activities, and he made sure we all knew how much we were loved. I prided myself during childhood on being a daddy's girl. I feel so lucky to have always had him by my side as my greatest mentor and for unconditional support.

My mom was an executive with Kaiser Permanente who had mastered work-life balance as a super-mom. She is as intelligent as driven, and my brother lucked out inheriting her brains and wit. She graduated top of her class in high school and was even offered a scholarship to Stanford but opted to stay closer to her small hometown in Arizona, attending college with her twin sister and brother at the University of Arizona in Tucson, where she later met my father. My mom is hands-down one of the most caring, patient, committed, generous-hearted, and loving people on the planet.

She is hardworking and highly successful at all she does. She always can, and will, do anything and everything for me, my brother, and my stepdad. We couldn't exist without her constant support. We are all so fortunate to have her close, and our bond through my becoming a parent has only brought us closer together. She is just as enthusiastic as a grandma and loves to let my kids explore and learn. They perform science experiments, such as pairing vinegar with baking soda to make exploding chalk bombs on her driveway. She takes the kids on muddy creek hikes, makes homemade ice cream and cookies, and spoils them with never-ending fun activities.

My dad had convinced my mom to move to San Francisco after they graduated from college, as he wanted to return closer to where he had grown up, just outside the city. After having my older brother, Scott, they decided to raise their growing family in the suburbs and moved just in time for my debut in life.

Their stark personality differences and the challenges of raising two young children ultimately led to the end of their marriage only a few short years after I was born. That turned out to be a win-win for everyone involved. Both of my parents are now happily remarried to their true life partners, who they are now growing old with all these years later.

I was also gifted with the world's greatest stepmom, who also had two kids by the time she met my father. So, I have bonus siblings: my little sister, Stacy, and older brother, Keith, who happened to be the same age and was a classmate of my older brother, Scott. Irene, my stepmom, helped raise me ever since coming into my life way back in the first grade. Along with her entire endearing family, she welcomed my brother and me into the fold with open arms and has always treated us as her very own. She coached my softball teams and treated all four of us kids with unconditional love. She did this all while working full time, juggling the chaos of our bustling, energetic home and parenting us four siblings with unending patience and ease. She was a fun mom who liked to play with us. I try to emulate her active and cool mom habits in my own life but fall far from her level of grace in mastering this challenge.

I've never liked using the word 'step' when talking about my family, especially when it comes to my stepsiblings. I blame Cinderella for adding a negative stigma to that title. My stepfamily has only proved to be a blessing of more love and has made life that much more beautiful an experience. Scott, Keith, Stacy, and I grew up happily together under the same roof and share a close bond. They are a big reason I had such a positive childhood, and I love them each with my entire heart.

During childhood, following our parents' divorce, Scott and I would move back and forth every Friday between our mom's and dad's houses, which were conveniently located less than a mile apart. My mom later married my stepfather, Courtney, who she met when I was in middle school. He has a daughter, Tori, my age, who lived with her mom and didn't move into our household. Tori has become a hip and fun-loving aunt to all my kids, and they love when she visits our family.

Courtney didn't enter our lives until my brother and I were pre-pubescent, know-it-all, protective-of-our-mother, tweens. He was also a little awkward adjusting to the newness of step-parental duties while dodging a lot of criticism from my brother and me. We were short-tempered and judgmental, thanks to our surging hormones. As a result, it took us a while longer to adapt to our family dynamic and the bond we now have today. Still, we became very close and have grown even closer since his and my mom's move to Southern California, bonding over his role as proud grandpa to my four kids.

My stepdad is quite an eclectic and impressive man. He was born and raised in Cambridge, Massachusetts, and later obtained both Master's and Doctorate degrees from Harvard. He has led an action-packed life as a civil rights activist, inspired by his father who was a highly respected Reverend and friend of Martin Luther King, Jr. Courtney was also an anti-war protester, refusing to serve as a soldier in Vietnam; instead, he chose to go to Vietnam to help heal the wounds of war. He was a volunteer with the American Friends Service Committee, working in a hospital where, during the TET offensive in 1968, he nearly lost his life while tirelessly working to save others. Upon coming home, he devoted his life to helping at-risk youth in gangs and later became active in politics. Recently, when he was invited to speak to Cristian and Sienna's 4th grade class during Martin Luther King week, he shared personal experiences from the 1965 civil rights movement... it was a moving and proud moment for us all.

All four of my parents have equally contributed to my becoming the complicated person I am today. As I always say, the more, the merrier. I was lucky to have been surrounded by love and support and turned out better off and more balanced in life because of their influences.

• • •

After the long week I had with the barrage of medical tests and high stress, I thanked my lucky stars. Finally, I could visit my mom and Courtney for some much-needed comfort while awaiting the biopsy and scan results.

It was late morning. I sat on their couch talking about how I didn't want to go through the entire weekend on edge. As if I had willed it to happen, moments later my phone started to ring. Dr. Dalal's name and phone number were brightly shining on the front of the cell phone screen.

My pulse was racing, and I faltered and fumbled as my hands shook while trying to answer the call, overwhelmed with nerves.

"Hello, this is Erin," I answered the phone.

"Hi, Erin. It's Dr. Dalal. I'm so sorry to have to tell you this. Really, I am. Calls like this are the worst part of my job and knowing that you have four young children makes this one that much more difficult. Your biopsy results have arrived, and I am afraid the mass has tested positive. You have cancer…."

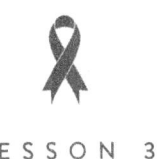

LESSON 3

Allow Yourself To Process The News

You have cancer. Hearing these three dreaded words spoken to you in real life feels much like you might imagine.

At first, I felt numb and emotionless. It seemed like I had taken a sucker punch to the gut leaving me unable to catch my breath. I distinctly recall my mom tightly squeezing my left hand with such force that I could feel my heart beating inside it.

I don't think she realized she was clinging onto me for dear life, but she was, and it hurt. It was distracting enough for me to know that the pain in my hand was as real as the conversation we were now having. This was happening.

Next, I became acutely focused on how my hand looked held inside of hers. I began to wonder how many times in life our two hands had held onto one another as they were in this moment. I could always reach out for her to take hold of me, and somehow this made me feel safe, secure, and protected. Holding onto my mom's hand always had a way of making everything seem right in the world.

I thought about the day that I was born and envisioned my baby fingers gently wrapping around hers for the very first time. I imagined how, at that moment, we likely formed the remarkable mother-daughter bond we still share today.

I noticed how our hands seemed so much older than they were from my early memories. Both of our hands are now covered in lines and weathered with signs of life. The instinct to grasp tightly onto one another in this dire moment seemed so natural.

I began to worry about what this must feel like for her. To bring a child into the world, raise and love them for 37 years, and then to suddenly have to process the heart-wrenching thought of losing them. She was holding herself together enough to speak with the doctor on my behalf, but I could see the fear behind her eyes. She was fighting back the tears.

My thoughts transitioned over to my own four children, and as soon as my husband and family entered my mind, the heavy emotion that accompanied this came crashing down and was more than I could bear. Tears began streaming down my cheeks, dripping from my chin and falling to my thighs, gently pooling on the tops of my purple leggings.

I must have dropped the phone at some point during the drama because my mom had hit the speakerphone and fully taken over the conversation that I had checked out from. I was unable to participate after entering a state of extreme shock. I could hear Dr. Dalal's voice on the line but can't recall much of what she said.

I could only take in small amounts of information and every so often would realize that my mom and Dr. Dalal were asking questions of me or repeating information to me to ensure that I was processing the most important takeaway points.

It is a drastic understatement to say discovering I had cancer felt like a cruel and devastating blow.

I started to fall into the various stages of grief, and then some. When the initial stage, Shock, began to fade, what came next was a process that, for me, went along the following trajectory.

Stage 2: Denial

It's not supposed to be this way. This kind of thing happened to other people. Not to me, and most certainly not now. I was in the middle of my life. This didn't seem fair. This form of a mid-life crisis was what happens in movies, dramatic stories with actors who portray a character for whom we come to feel a tremendous sense of loss and sadness.

I've seen this scene play out many times before. I often imagined what I would do if that ever happened to me in my own life. And then I'd feel a sense of relief, remembering that this was a tragic story about someone else.

Except on this day, it was happening to me and in real life. It is like being wide awake during your worst nightmare and pinching your arm to awaken from the bad dream. Only you come to realize that no matter how desperately you try to wake yourself up, nothing you do will make this go away.

Stage 3: Anger
Once reality started to settle in, a strange sense of anger followed the state of denial. This emotion rather surprised me because I'm not usually a very pessimistic or angry person. These emotions felt unfamiliar and were noticeable because of that.

I pent up a lot of anger for several days. Emotional baggage would bubble to the surface during the most unusual of circumstances. I would find myself feeling jealous of strangers for no reason other than that they had their health and seemed to take it for granted.

I'd see someone driving on the road through the window of their car, seemingly without a care in the world. I'd suddenly feel a sense of envy over them for not having to worry about problems as extreme as a matter of life or death. I wanted to switch bodies with them.

As soon as I took enough time to examine this bizarre reaction more closely, I identified the root cause for my anger as stemming from the question, "Why me?" Why not that guy who cut me off in traffic, putting my family and several other cars in danger while having the audacity to flip us all the bird? He seemed like an authentic jerk and was way more deserving of cancer. What was happening to me felt so unfair, disproportionate, and I was furious about it.

I had gone to the car line at the kids' school to pick them up the week after my diagnosis. I was having a superficial conversation trying to make small talk with a mom I had only just met.

She was rambling on to me about her frustration over her current kitchen remodel. Her contractor had shown up more than an hour late that morning, causing her to miss an important appointment she had scheduled.

When she returned home after running errands, she discovered her kitchen was destroyed. The contractor was long gone and had not cleaned up the demolition clutter before leaving for the weekend. The mess was left for her to rummage through, and she was short-tempered over the growing inconvenience the home remodel was causing her to suffer.

She arrived at school already annoyed and fuming over how the school bus returning the kids from their field trip was running late, stuck in Friday rush hour traffic. The class had been visiting a museum in Los Angeles, and now her entire afternoon schedule was going to need to be adjusted accordingly, and her poor son likely would be late to his soccer practice. What a bad day she was having.

Around this point in the conversation, she finally paused to catch her breath and looked up to find me blankly staring back at her. That must have caught her off guard, and she reacted by taking a moment to extend the common courtesy of asking me how my day was going.

What I wanted to tell her was, "Do you have any clue how fortunate you are that these are the problems keeping you up at night? Your greatest concern in life is the inconvenience of a kitchen renovation. I would give anything to trade places with you. You don't have any idea as to what real problems are."

What I said instead was the expected response of, "Fine, thanks for asking."

I bit my tongue and rolled my eyes while fuming on the inside. I knew she didn't deserve my anger and judgment, but I was mad at life and the world. My visceral thoughts were that I was starting to become rather jaded and cynical.

The strange part about being diagnosed with cancer is that there is no one to be angry with. It wasn't anyone's fault. The poor people onto whom I was projecting my fury were innocent bystanders at the wrong place, at the wrong time, happening to be standing in my line of fire.

Had the school mom and I had this very same conversation only a couple of weeks prior, I likely would have supported her frustrations over the inconvenience. But standing in my newfound identity as a cancer patient made these things seem like small problems—temporary and minor setbacks in the grand scheme of life. I wished I, too, could be oblivious enough to worry over the small stuff in place of the shit storm I found myself standing in.

Cancer has a way of quickly cutting through the bullshit. You recognize that allowing ourselves to get so easily worked up over many things is just us sweating the small stuff. Most of our problems are indeed just small stuff.

I had an epiphany that day while in conversation with the school mom. It allowed me to suddenly see how many of the dilemmas over which I used to consume myself were, most often, not worth the weight I gave them.

Real problems, the big ones, inevitably do occur in life, and when this happens, we need to process all the heavy emotions they carry. This is perfectly normal and also very necessary. If you are mad, get mad. So long as you eventually recognize the negative emotions you feel and catch yourself when you start spiraling down the rabbit hole.

At which point you need to ask yourself the following question: "Is this problem going to exist or still impact me five years from today?"

If the answer is no, then my rule of thumb is it isn't worth your fretting over for more than five minutes. Doing that is a waste of your valuable time and energy. It can be categorized as an issue that falls under 'small stuff.'

That may sound easier said than done, I know. When the answer to the above question is yes, a similar rule applies. The bigger problems that will impact you in the long term, such as a cancer diagnosis, for example, should get no more than three to five days' attention before you need to crash in on your pity party.

You are allowed more time when talking about the big stuff like divorce, loss of a job, grieving a lost loved one, or chronic disease. Big problems like these still have a shelf life, though, in terms of how long you should allow yourself to wallow in them.

You can certainly allow extra time for processing the real problems in life, but be mindful over how long you allow yourself to remain in this dangerous place. Staying down in the dumps is a dangerous space to be for too long. For the big stuff, try to stick to three to five days. You may not be over it by this point, but you should be able to have lifted yourself out of being stuck in your state of despair by that time.

It is often said that energy flows where attention goes. Unless you want more grief in your own life, eventually you will need to snap out of it and move forward. Staying in any negative state of mind for too long will only attract further suffering, keeping you stuck in a vicious cycle of wallowing in your pity which can eventually become dangerous for your health.

As for my case, as terrible as the cancer diagnosis was, I realized the time had come for my alter ego, a.k.a. Debbie Downer, to be evicted. I saw how I was caught in an angry, sad, and confused space. After realizing this, I decided the time had come to pick myself up, dry my tears, put one foot in front of the other, and try hard to start moving forward as best I could.

You are still allowed to have bad days, especially during a season of life that comes with something as drastic as a permanent life change. Real-life big problems hurt, and you won't get over them quickly. Just don't stay down in the dumps long enough to make this your new normal or allow your crisis to cause more damage than necessary.

The anger phase can leave you feeling invincible, whereas the next phase of sadness leaves you feeling exposed. Anger and sadness are common reactions to a negative experience where something important to you feels like it has been wronged. And it's easy for one emotion to take the place of the other, depending on your naturally triggered defensive response.

Both emotions offer you the chance to make sense of a bad situation, but the phases experienced as you work your way through them are very different.

When I was angry, I had built up walls and prepared to go to battle. I was ready to go on the attack and was easily triggered. What I had needed was comfort, patience, and time to process this awkward phase fully. I honestly think it may have been easier to be angry than it was to be sad. Maybe that is why the anger phase often comes before the sadness?

Stage 4: Sadness
Anger gets you fired up. It is an active emotion, whereas sadness is a passive one. Sadness makes you feel raw and vulnerable. It leaves you to feel the full pain and all the hurt that you have just sustained. I don't think this part of the process can happen until you have grown weary of the rage.

Of course I was sad. I needed to allow myself time to grieve the changes that were happening. Like missing out on the holiday season that I wished I could be preparing for instead of dealing with cancer.

The week after Thanksgiving, I was supposed to take down the pilgrims and turkey decor and start putting up festive holiday lights. This is when our family goes in search of finding the perfect Christmas tree. It's when we take the kids to see Santa and begin shopping for presents for friends and family members. We usually pen countless holiday parties for work and friends and school performances onto our calendar. This was supposed to be a joyful season. A time where, in my role as a wife and mother, I usually get to create magic for those I love. I typically pride myself on selecting the perfect family photo to feature on our Season's Greeting card, but this year needed one that read "We Wish You a Merry Cancer Christmas and Tragic New Year."

I wanted to attend my kids' winter recitals, not go to my pre-op appointments. We did attempt to attend church for the holidays, which turned out to be an utter disaster. That was way too daunting an experience that I was not ready for. The children's choir was performing Christmas songs at this service, and I was overwhelmed with a deep sense of sorrow that I couldn't process in public view.

As I watched the kids up on the stage, I reminisced about singing in holiday performances during my own childhood. I looked at the sweet faces of my innocent children and thought about how depressing it was that this could be my last Christmas alive.

The grim reality led to a massive panic attack. I couldn't sit in the pew long enough for the song to finish and had to abruptly trip over people to exit the sanctuary so that I could bolt to the bathroom, slam the stall door behind me, and sit on top of a toilet fully dressed in my best church attire while sobbing into mounds of toilet paper. It was way too much, too soon. More than my tender heart could handle.

It's normal to be deeply sad about a cancer diagnosis, especially as a young adult, and even more so as a parent.

I didn't want to die. Maybe the hardest part to cope with in the sadness phase was whenever I had to think about how this would impact my children. That made me feel depressed beyond measure. I didn't want to miss out on the many joys and milestones in their lives or the parental love and honor I was supposed to experience as a privilege of being their proud mom.

Nor did I want my own life to end long before I even had the chance to live my fair share of it. I had ignorantly always assumed that the years that lay ahead were a given. The gift of life and time experiencing it wasn't supposed to end this soon. I grieved over my life often and felt unspeakable sadness over the thought of my death.

Going through treatment for cancer doesn't help in the sadness arena either. It's hard to be cheerful while being nauseous, tired, or suffering in physical pain from the common side effects of treatment. Just like that, instantaneously, I had lost all sense of normalcy in life as I knew it. This stage was hard.

I grieved over the loss of myself and my life. Sadness has a way of creeping in early, repeatedly, and often throughout cancer. A cancer diagnosis hurts deeply. Just as with anger, sadness is an uncomfortable feeling that you will have to allow yourself to sit in and feel.

Doing this is not easy. I didn't know it at the time but learning to process all the intense negative emotions of shock, denial, anger, and sadness was a life lesson I needed to master on my road to recovery. I had never allowed myself to fully experience uncomfortable emotions long enough to feel them so deeply that I could process through them and finally analyze them objectively.

I had a habit of quickly brushing aside whatever I didn't like to feel, often burying pain and discomfort internally before moving along as quickly as possible. I somehow understood, however, that during this process of grief following my cancer diagnosis, I needed to do things differently from what I was accustomed to. I instinctively understood that this would come to serve an integral role in my recovery. And so, instead of avoiding the difficult phases, I developed a deep connection to myself, went inward, and embraced them all.

During sadness, I grieved deeply. The most I could do with the sadness was recognize it as something I needed to face, feel, and process as a step in the right direction. The hard truth is that emotions like anger and sadness will come to play a very important part in your journey to living beyond cancer.

I told myself that maybe this time next year, if I am lucky enough to still be alive, the sadness will have probably gotten easier. During this stage, something that helped me start my day was focusing on what was working well in my life. The many things that I had to be grateful for.

I cuddled and hugged my kids often. I held onto them a little tighter and a while longer than I had before. I told my husband every single morning just how much I loved and appreciated him. I called my parents and my siblings more often and thanked them for all our happy memories, or just to let them know how much I loved them too.

I eventually came to discover that gratitude has a way of helping heal sadness. Giving thanks for the people and things in life that you feel appreciative for can be incredibly cathartic. It is healing and has a way of easing the burden of pain.

Stage 5: Hypothetical Questions

This is the stage where I started to ask myself many 'what if' statements and considered an infinite number of possibilities. If only I had done X differently, maybe this never would have happened. I reflected a lot over what had transpired in my life before the day of my diagnosis. Four months had passed from the onset of symptoms. The tumor in my colon had grown to be two inches in size.

I couldn't help but question how things might be different if only I had been diagnosed sooner. What if I could have even avoided cancer altogether? Countless hypothetical scenarios swirled through my head.

All of my doctors seemed stumped over my diagnosis. I wasn't overweight. My recent physical exam months prior showed I was the epitome of health, other than being very anemic. I was an avid runner and appeared to be in peak physical condition.

I was too young and had no family history of cancer. None of my parents, aunts, or uncles have had cancer. My grandmother had breast cancer later in her life, and my grandfather passed from pancreatic cancer in his seventies, but neither of those seemed to explain why I had developed colorectal cancer at 37 years old. Genetic testing would later prove I had no predisposition for developing cancer.

Of course, there's no point in lingering over the mystery behind this diagnosis. The many hypothetical theories, the many 'what ifs' and 'if onlys' will keep you up at night. Each doctor who told me that my case didn't make sense made it only more discouraging. They all said that I didn't fit the list of usual suspects. While I appreciated their telling me how healthy I ought to be, not one doctor could answer the questions that haunted me most. The frustration from this only seemed to make matters worse.

These are questions I may never receive a definitive answer for. I realized that fretting over them wasn't doing me any favors.

I had cancer. It happened. Time to deal with it.

When I was finished fretting over the many hypothetical theories, I was finally ready to seek answers to the hard questions. Like how did I get here? Why did this happen? Now that I'm here, what should I do about it? Where do I go from this point?

I wanted to know. Heck, if cancer was going to take me down, I needed to make some sense out of it. I think it is part of human nature to try and find meaning or make sense of life. And so, I set out on a mission to seek answers, which is a perfect transition into the next stage of the post-cancer-diagnosis process.

Stage 6: Knowledge Seeker

I grabbed every book, scoured through countless websites and blogs, listened to podcasts, and sifted through medical reports and journals to learn how this could have happened. I was an information-seeking machine on a path to understanding everything there is to know about cancer.

I discovered so much I wished I had known before being diagnosed, including steps I could have taken to reduce my risk of ever developing it. I learned the dangerous mistakes I had been making that I have since come to believe likely contributed to my illness. I also identified how best to care for myself now that I had cancer to treat and wanted to survive it.

I consumed a lot of information and research and did so in a relatively short time frame. I didn't have the luxury of time on my side, so this phase is what I often refer to as the crash course in Cancer 101.

I also noticed there was a repetitive theme in almost every one of the cancer resources I studied. I discovered recurring themes that many cancer survivors and doctors attribute to increasing odds of survival and decided to apply them to my health action plan. In one such book that I lovingly refer to as my cancer bible, *Radical Remission: Surviving Cancer Against All Odds,* Dr. Kelly A. Turner, founder of the Radical Remission Project, uncovers nine factors that she says can lead to a spontaneous remission from cancer—even after conventional medicine has failed.

That book and website include thousands of first-hand testimonials from cancer patients who went on to live long, fulfilling lives long after they had been deemed too sick to cure and were not expected to survive. Many are stories of those who were sent home on hospice care that later went on to enjoy the remainder of a life well-lived years into their old age. It gave me hope that I could chase the same results.

Stage 7: Acceptance

Acceptance by no means is letting go of or ignoring the emotions you need to experience to work your way through this. At least for me, acceptance was coming to a place of simply being at peace with all of it.

I had reached the point where I was ready to put all my energy towards surviving whatever was to come—not just surviving it but thriving through it. Learning to appreciate every setback, bump in the road and the painful and often uncomfortable parts of the journey.

I knew that I was going into the fight of my life, and there came a point where I realized wasting precious time in denial, feeling angry, sad, victimized, and confused was not doing me any favors.

I still have moments or days when extreme emotions return. Whenever this happens, I now recognize this as an identifiable phase of a process that I now know how to navigate my way through. After I finished working my way through the many emotions and phases experienced following my diagnosis, I learned how to accept my reality and move forward with the set intention of living whatever life I had left to the fullest.

I am a runner, and my oncologist, after we first met, told me to think of cancer treatment as my greatest marathon. Fair warning, this is indeed going to be a marathon to work your way through, not a sprint. It's full of twists, turns, unexpected challenges, triumphs and victories; and discovery of how strong you never realized you are until forced to push yourself to your limits and greatest test. It's going to take time to navigate the course. We all know that anything worth chasing after never comes easily. In the end, you will discover that every uphill battle offers a valuable takeaway that you can grow through and use for good.

I worked my way through processing every phase above during my cancer journey, and when I finished treatment continued to learn and grow through what this experience has brought into my life.

I promised that whatever new setbacks come my way, no matter how devastating the news, the inevitable loss, the challenges, and the pain, I trust that I am capable of processing more than I ever realized. You, too, will fail forward, and you will also fall. The key is to rise back up, dry those tears, brush yourself off, and keep placing one foot in front of the other, moving forward one step at a time.

I realized that to survive cancer, I would need to find courage, strength, and acceptance to use cancer as my greatest opportunity for growth. Cancer was part of my story, whether I liked it or not. I accepted that, and in doing so, regained a sense of control to face it wholeheartedly.

To get through it, I needed to own it. Accepting my cancer diagnosis was the hardest thing I've ever had to overcome in all my life. I decided to view it as a brief passing moment in time, a season of my greater life, rather than a persistent state of being that I couldn't live beyond.

This would never have been placed before me if it wasn't something I was born capable of enduring. Living beyond my cancer diagnosis was my new life purpose, and I would use it to get wherever this experience was meant to take me.

Stage 8: Cancer Warrior & Fighter

I don't always like how people refer to those living with or who have survived cancer as warriors and fighters.

These two terms are commonly associated with cancer patients and are titles I admit I initially struggled with. I see the irony because I named this book after being a mother and a cancer fighter.

Yes, as a cancer patient, I was preparing for the greatest battle in my life, but I'm not a fighter by nature, and the analogy didn't feel like a suitable one for me. I didn't embrace it, at least not at first.

The final phase of discovering my cancer-fighter mentality didn't hit home until shortly after reaching the acceptance phase. It was my way of taking ownership over having cancer. I finally came to terms with this as part of my story and decided that I was ready to reclaim whatever control I could hold over my diagnosis and live a life beyond this. That is when the true Mother Fighter inside of me stepped into this story.

A group of friends from my daughter's softball team, coincidentally named The Warriors, gave me a beautiful gift while I was recovering in the hospital following my surgery. It was a silver bracelet with an inspirational quote inscribed on the inside of the band.

"Fate whispers to the warrior, 'You cannot withstand the storm.' The warrior whispers back, 'I am the storm.'"

I greatly appreciated the kind gesture and also the idea of finally embracing my warrior mentality.

It's about finding the courage inside of yourself to do something harder than you believe you are capable of. More importantly, do this even when you don't feel like it. Face the big stuff you would prefer not to deal with at all, the stuff it would be much easier to ignore or avoid if this weren't a matter of life and death.

•••

I have a confession to share. Before becoming a cancer warrior, I was a self-professed wimp. If I had been given a choice, I most certainly would have tapped out of this fight against cancer. When friends and family told me how brave they thought I was, I felt like an imposter. I was a fake who was undeserving of a glorious title such as courageous fighter and warrior.

When I think of people I consider to be brave, do you know who comes to mind?

Real heroes whose lives had a massive influence on others and who have changed the world. People like Nelson Mandela, Rosa Parks, Malala Yousafzai, Oprah Winfrey, and Martin Luther King Jr. People who came face-to-face with life-altering adversity. They stood up for something greater than themselves, for a cause to end suffering or a much-needed effort for change. I can think of many I would deem worthy of the hard-earned title "hero." They are inspirational.

I, however, never felt comfortable or deserving when hearing those words spoken about little ol' me. I am none of those things. I just happened to have cancer and did what was needed to do to survive it. The same thing you likely would have done were you put in the same situation. I would never have willingly volunteered to be in this position. I didn't have a choice.

Whenever someone asks me what I do, my answer always is that I do whatever it takes. If doing that makes me inspirational in some way, I guess I'll own it.

I ultimately realized that others saw me in this light even if I was unwilling to embrace being viewed as courageous, despite it making me squirm with discomfort. Which meant I had to take some responsibility for it even if I didn't fully believe it for myself. This encouraged me to raise the bar in my own life, to live up to the high expectation and perseverance others saw in me. I had to get to work on my recovery. It was time to fight for my life.

I Hope This Helps

When people hear my story, I am often asked whether I experienced symptoms prior to my diagnosis. The answer to that question is yes; however, symptoms are only one of what I consider a three-point essential information list about colon cancer. Knowing all three could help save your life:

- » Cancer is on the rise in young adults
- » It's best to be tested for colon cancer before symptoms are experienced
- » Knowing the symptoms of colon cancer will help you seek treatment

Cases of colon cancer are on the rise in young adults and the median age of patients diagnosed is getting lower. The disease is rising at alarming rates in people ages 18 to 35 and half of all new diagnoses this year will be in people under the age of 66.[1]

One article I recently read reported that if the current trends continue, by 2030 colon cancer cases are projected to increase by 90% in patients under age 35, and rectal cancer cases are expected to increase by 124% in this young patient age range.[2]

My mysterious onset of cancer proved to be more than a case of extremely bad luck. What I discovered was that there are far too many stories similar to my own. I am just one of many young adults who have become part of the new normal in a dangerous colorectal cancer trend that everyone needs to pay closer attention to.

You would be surprised at how many parents with children are members of the colorectal cancer support groups that I joined. The sheer numbers stunned me.

I recognized there is a critical need to inform, educate and raise awareness around this disease.

People are dying because people aren't talking about the symptoms that we all need to look out for. People don't understand how critical it is to inquire about screening should they have any symptoms. My goal is to change that and to share what others need to know in order to protect their health.

Maybe the most frightening part about colon cancer is how easy it is to dismiss the common symptoms that many cancer patients exhibit. In many cases, people who have these symptoms do not have cancer, but you should still talk to your doctor if you have any of them in order for the cause to be found and treated. It is advised that you contact your doctor if you have any of the following problems.[3]

COLON CANCER SIGNS & SYMPTOMS

- A change in bowel habits, such as diarrhea, constipation, or narrowing of the stool, which lasts for more than a few days
- A feeling that you need to have a bowel movement that's not relieved by having one
- Rectal bleeding with bright red blood
- Blood in the stool, which might make the stool look dark brown or black
- Cramping or abdominal (belly) pain
- Weakness and fatigue
- Unintended weight loss

In hindsight, I had every symptom on the above list. Their onset started months prior to my diagnosis. They persisted but were not distressing enough for me to seek medical attention until after it was too late.

Colorectal cancer is sometimes referred to as the "silent killer" because it often doesn't cause symptoms until after it has grown or spread. This year in the United States, 52,980 people are expected to die of the disease and 147,950 cases of colon cancer will be diagnosed.

It is the second most common cause of cancer deaths when men and women are combined. It is also one of the most preventable.[4]

The one thing I really want everyone to know is that you should start screening for colorectal cancer no later than the age of 45 even if you aren't experiencing any symptoms. Sooner, if you are experiencing any of the signs above or have a family history.

When found early through screening, it can be easier to treat. Screening can even prevent some colon cancers by finding and removing pre-cancerous growths called polyps.

While writing this book, the recommended age to begin screening was lowered to age 45 due to the increase in cases among younger people. What is most frightening is that, when many young adults are diagnosed with colorectal cancer, it is with advanced Stages 3 and 4, when it's more difficult to treat. I am a prime example of this frightening statistic.

According to the latest trends, 1 in 3 people in the U.S. will be diagnosed with cancer in their lifetime. More than 1.8 million new cases of cancer are expected to be diagnosed in the U.S. alone this year.[5] There are a variety of reasons believed to contribute to the rise of cancer rates in young adults. We'll cover more on these topics as we proceed in the chapters to come.

As an advocate using my story to inform others about cancer, my goal is to educate and point out the importance of early detection. It's to spark the conversation we all need to be having and to raise awareness in an effort to help others. There are steps you can take today if you are sick, or just looking to protect yourself and those you love, by learning habits of wellness and prevention.

PART II

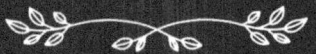

How to Heal
the Mind

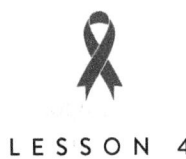

LESSON 4

CANCER IS A SYMPTOM, FIND THE SOURCE

SOS is a morse code distress signal originally established for maritime use. It is often used in phrases such as 'Save Our Souls' and 'Save Our Ship.' The saying has come to indicate a moment of crisis or need for action. Following my cancer diagnosis, I felt like I was standing on a sinking ship. That day was unquestionably an example of a moment of crisis requiring the immediate need for action.

What you don't know is that the ship I had been standing on had been sinking for years, long before the day of my diagnosis. That pivotal moment was merely the tidal wave that came crashing down, delivering the final blow that ultimately sank the vessel. I had been desperately clinging to that vessel for dear life, sending out a distress signal for help that had yet to be answered. The day had finally arrived where the ship sunk to the bottom of the sea, and now all that was left to do was raise a white flag and surrender.

I believe all that had transpired leading up to that day played a critical role in contributing to my cancer diagnosis.

This chapter was not an easy one for me to write. To tell you what happened, I must first let you in on a family secret. This will require exposing some scary skeletons in the back of the closet that were never intended for others to see. It is something that many of our closest friends and family members were not even aware of.

I questioned how vulnerable I should be in discussing my personal life in this book when writing this chapter. These are things my husband and I made an intentional effort to hide. We did an admirable job at keeping these matters private. Sharing it here for the world to read seems a bit counterintuitive. Still, I now know that burying this part of our life away from sight, internalizing the pain, and suppressing the emotional toll this carried with it had a very negative impact on my health.

Airing our dirty laundry in a book is difficult to do, but I see value in including this because I know others experiencing similar struggles in their own lives might gain strength by my sharing this part of my story and learning how I worked through it. This is a book about overcoming a life crisis, after all. While I intend to keep the topic around my story with cancer, this needs to be discussed as I believe it relates to my developing the disease and could have even been a root cause behind it. It was also because of cancer that I ultimately was able to sort through these debilitating issues that I had failed to overcome in the years before.

My husband and I mastered putting out a facade that all was well when, in reality, behind the walls of our home we had been drowning in a sea of insurmountable financial debt as a result of legal troubles. The two naturally go hand-in-hand, but the point is we have been surviving in a chronic state of intense stress for the last eight very long and painful years. That's a long time to struggle. Too long, dangerously long. And it took a drastic toll on my health.

•••

Our money troubles began in 2008. We all remember what happened to the economy that year after the market crashed, pushing our country into recession. Will is in the real estate industry, and his job took a massive hit, but that wasn't the factor that catapulted us into extreme debt. It was unfortunate real estate investments on residential and commercial properties that sealed our fate. He lost everything in his name trying to realize a dream that would come to haunt us for years to come.

His commercial investment was an emotional purchase brought about by his ambition, with the best of intentions, to emulate his parents' footsteps. Will was born in Los Angeles in 1976. His parents had come to the United States, relocating from Mexico, young, eager, and ambitious, to chase their American dream.

They became citizens, grew a family with three children, and worked incredibly hard to build a business. They represent the epitome of the classic entrepreneurial success story. The Sotos started with one, which then became several, taco trucks while living in a tiny apartment in East Los Angeles. Their taco truck business grew into a restaurant. Will's mother, Catalina, raised their three children in a beautiful house with a pool in Downey, California when their marriage ended. She was, still is, one of the greatest chefs to ever walk the planet. She also is one of the most generous-hearted and hard-working women I know.

She practically lived at Soto's Restaurant, eventually buying out her husband and building a booming business that fans of her food would travel long distances to enjoy. She worked at the restaurant tirelessly, sprinkling plenty of love into her craft until her retirement. Soto's Restaurant is now called something else, but the building and memories from Will's childhood all remain.

Will grew up with his parents' example of how hard work can pay off in achieving your dreams, resulting in tremendous success. They took a chance moving to a new and foreign country, barely speaking the language so many years before. Becoming American citizens with a hard-earned and wild success story continues to impress the generations of Soto family who follow. Will learned to speak English only after he started kindergarten; he grew up a true California child of the eighties and a proud member of Generation X.

I often catch him reminiscing over the good ol' days, jamming to his questionable choices in music and favorite classic movies. He is six years my senior and loves to remind me that I can't claim to be one of the Gen X cool kids as I technically am one of the oldest members of the highly criticized Millennials. Will's childhood wasn't always easy, but he was raised with love and had many friends. He thrived at Catholic schools and sports and surfed the waters of Malibu, spritzing Sun-In for beachy streaks in his long hair. After first attending college at Pepperdine University, he later graduated from California State University, Fullerton.

Will has always been committed to actualizing the entrepreneurial spirit his parents inspired in him during childhood. When the neighbor who owned the commercial building filling the other half of the block next to Soto's Restaurant proposed to Will that he partner with him, he accepted, appreciating this as an opportunity to begin his own commercial property investment. The property held several small businesses, including a dry cleaner and florist. The neighbor was Will's parents' age; he hoped to retire soon. He chose to approach my husband knowing that the Soto family might well be interested in eventually owning the entire city block. When things sound too good to be true, often this is because they are.

Will trusted him and poured every penny to his name, his life savings of more than half a million dollars, into what would prove to be a terrible investment for a property that never stood a chance to begin with. He should have walked away. More like run in the other direction and never look back, but he didn't. This investment would later prove to be one of the greatest and most costly mistakes of our family's life. The building was old and in such a state of disrepair by the time Will entered the equation that he would soon lose all he had poured into this doomed investment. He'd given more and more until there was nothing left to give

Around the same time the commercial property flopped, so did the residential flip we had taken on when I was pregnant with the twins. The house flip was supposed to help us earn back some of what we had lost from the commercial flop. It was a desperate attempt that plummeted along with home values in late 2008.

The debt we now owed after both investments tanked was in the hundreds of thousands of dollars. We did the only thing we could think of to survive, which was short selling our townhome, packing up our newborn babies, and moving in with my mother-in-law to start over from scratch.

We couldn't even afford to rent our own place. If we were going to dig ourselves out of the mountain of debt we had accumulated, we needed first to sacrifice privacy and move in with Will's mom during this difficult time. We accepted her generous offer to help save on the cost of housing, and we both got to work paying off debt and saving every cent to our name with the hope of buying our own home again someday in the future.

Isn't it ironic how some of our toughest breaks will simultaneously coincide with the greatest of life's miracles? Our newborn twins and the joy we had from our growing family bond were just the glimmers of hope needed to get us both through that difficult time.

Our temporary living arrangement was challenging, but it would come to offer us several blessings. The first was that our twins received an enormity of love poured over them by their Abuela while we were off and away at work. One couldn't ask for better care, and they were spoiled and cherished beyond measure. The next blessing was that I got to enjoy eating all of her delicious food! I even learned how to recreate some of her most beloved famous dishes but, to this day, I will never live up to her natural talent and gift in the kitchen. I'm drooling as I type, just thinking about Abuela's cooking now.

We wanted to give our twins the world and were driven to do whatever it took to recuperate from the financial loss and land back on our feet, for their sake more than our own. Parenthood was a welcome respite that gave us the energy and willpower needed to muster through the course of the next five years while we both worked diligently to rebuild our livelihood.

We put our heads down, worked hard, and focused on the goal of buying ourselves a future family home. It took us five years to reach that endpoint. We had paid off most of our debt and slowly but surely scraped up just enough savings for the down payment. With the help of my mom and a family friend generously lending us the last needed funds to complete our purchase, in 2013 we were finally able to buy what was supposed to be our family's forever home.

We moved to San Juan Capistrano just in time to celebrate the first birthday of our third child, Taylor. We were house poor but proud homeowners, and after everything we had been through to earn that title, it left us feeling like we were standing on top of the world. We had big dreams to restore and fix up our broken, run-down house, grand plans to perfect every nook and cranny while we raised our growing family in it.

•••

Just as we took that milestone step forward, we were unexpectedly thrust right back, knocking us arguably to the lowest of all lows, far down to the very bottom again. Not even 30 days after moving into our house, the business partner from the commercial investment all those years prior decided to sue my husband over a disagreement about the property. Will was caught completely off guard, as so many years had passed without any inclination that his former partner held grievances against him. You can imagine our sincere surprise when faced with a lawsuit asking Will to pay him approximately a million dollars! We can only imagine the reasoning behind this lawsuit, but the timing certainly seemed rather more than coincidental. Perhaps he had falsely assumed we had equity in the house we'd just bought and ample money to spare?

Maybe he sadly blamed my husband for their drastic and unfortunate loss over their investment? As if we hadn't already lost enough right along with him when the property tanked. What hurt more was that this was someone Will had trusted. The only difference now was that we had since worked to pull ourselves up and out following the devastation, and it seemed as though he hated seeing our family succeed. Of course, this reflects my recollection of this experience, and conclusions are based on my opinion.

We were naive to believe that justice would prevail and refused to agree to a settlement. This case seemed frivolous, malicious even, and we trusted knowing the truth to defend ourselves. We hoped this would eventually end peacefully. We believed our innocence would protect us. Considering how the entire case was based upon a disagreement over the property, with many false accusations that lacked any proof for the alleged claims, we honestly didn't think it could succeed. I regret sharing that our rose-colored lens, believing that the good guys will prevail, has sadly been jaded.

The financial and mental impact that lawsuits cause to those who bear their burden extends over into your relationships, touching upon every aspect of your personal life. During the worst of times, throughout this tumultuous situation, our marriage began to suffer over the pain experienced from the inability to provide for our family financially.

As young parents trying to raise what grew to be four young children, desperate to save our hard bought house and keep a roof over their heads, clothes on their bodies and food in their tummies, the need to continually pay out offensive sums of legal defense expenses harmed us substantially. It was no small feat.

I grew accustomed to living under financial strain and perfected my shocked response whenever my grocery store declined my debit card. I was reminded of our insufficient funds the many times this happened but would act as though it had come as a complete surprise.

More times than I care to admit I had to abandon full shopping carts, assuring clerks I'd soon return to complete my purchase after a quick call to the bank to investigate the mystery behind why my card was not functioning. I, of course, never went back, but instead cried after safely hiding in the privacy of my car, feeling defeated.

Speaking of our car, the family minivan was repossessed on several occasions, twice while parked outside of my husband's office. Talk about embarrassing. One time this happened while my husband was on his way out of the office to pick up the kids from school. This left us scrambling to find a friend to safely watch our children while we drove an hour away to reclaim our vehicle from the repo lot it had been towed to.

We maxed out all our credit cards, and when those limits were reached, we progressed to using my mom's cards and maxing out hers as well. She even took out an equity line on her own home just to keep us afloat. Do you know what it feels like to be a grown adult with children of your own still living off the support of your retired parents on a fixed income?

Every time we swallowed our pride and resorted to asking for help from family, it was the worst feeling of utter failure. The last thing my husband and I wanted was to be dependent on our parents. We were lucky to have some family willing to help us cover the kids' cost to play soccer or softball, and to help pay a month's mortgage in order to keep our house.

Will worked tirelessly, earning more than enough to cover our mortgage and the cost of living, but the onslaught of attorney bills, at $10,000 a pop every month or two for so many years, proved to be more than we could muster. We had somehow accumulated debt again into the hundreds of thousands of dollars due to legal expenses, and this time there was no end in sight or a way to work ourselves out of the hardship we were drowning in.

The lawsuit was the gift that kept on taking, robbing us of our ability to survive. We paid our attorney instead of buying the kids much-needed shoes, winter jackets, and groceries. The dreams of remodeling our home never got off to a start because the attorney fees piled in before we had even finished unpacking the moving boxes.

That season was a never-ending vicious cycle of living paycheck to paycheck while falling further behind into tremendous debt.

•••

I worried for my husband's health, who over the years had several near heart attacks from the stress he was under to provide for the family.

In the summer before my cancer diagnosis, I started experiencing severe panic attacks, with one so intense that it involved a nervous breakdown requiring strong medication and someone to intervene in helping care for the kids for several days until I could pull myself up from the pain. My full-blown mental meltdown happened just six months before my cancer diagnosis. It was also just before the majority of my cancer symptoms suddenly emerged. I see more than coincidence in that timing.

Before the worst of that extreme attack happened, I had come home from dropping the kids off at school to find Will sitting at the foot of our bed. His eyes were bloodshot, and he looked like a broken, fragile, grief-stricken man who had reached the end of his line.

Will has only cried a handful of times over the 17 years we have been together. Seeing him in this state on that morning scared the living daylights out of me. He was nearly suicidal and told me he felt like he had failed me as a husband, couldn't provide for our children as their father, and was a disappointment as a son, brother, and person.

In his eyes he was a failure, felt worthless, and even had questioned whether his life was cursing those he loved most. He told me he had nothing left to give and believed that the world and our family might be better off without him in it. The most frightening part about this conversation was how he meant the insane words that he was speaking. It was terrifying and broke my heart right along with his own.

My husband is one of the most generous-hearted, honest, and good-natured people I've ever met. He is a man of the utmost integrity. He quite literally has taken the shirt off his back to give to another. Countless friends, family, and colleagues who know him love to share story upon story about what an upstanding person he is and the times he went the extra mile to help others. That said, you can understand why the painful allegations that were being made, viciously attacking his character, that we knew to be untrue and seemingly coming from out of nowhere, hurt him deeply.

The mortgage was months overdue, and we were very close to losing the home. The house we had fought so hard to keep over the years after buying it with so many dreams. Our one goal throughout the legal nightmare had always been to save the house for the kids. If only we could keep them in the comfort of their familiar home. It was our way of protecting them from having to bear the brunt of catastrophic ramifications this lawsuit caused our family.

Our home was unfurnished, broken, and in desperate need of repair, but it was still their home. It was their haven from the outside world. We did our very best to hide how bad things had become from the kids. We put on a brave face and outward surface appearance that all was well. We attempted to keep the kids feeling protected and untouched by the chaos that we were experiencing. They had glimpses of it, though, and we couldn't hide it from them entirely.

The pivotal day of my mental breakdown would prove to be a turning point in our family's life. The time had come for us to finally surrender, out of having no fight left inside and our growing too tired of swimming upstream. We were mentally exhausted from surviving in a state of constant desperation. We were ready to raise the white flag and take action for unwelcome and extremely uncomfortable but necessary change. We agreed that neither of us could live another day as we had been and that we needed to acknowledge we had hit rock bottom.

I sat down on the floor beside Will that morning and grabbed his hands in mine, pleading with him not to give up on us. While this lawsuit seemed to be based on a mission to take away our livelihood, the one thing it could never steal from us is the core of what matters most. Our family. Our love for one another.

For better or worse, we were going to get through this. I knew it. We were going to do it together. We had to remain strong and persevere for our children who needed us to succeed. We had a lot of love between us all, and that was what had gotten us this far. We had each other. We had our health. Things could always be worse, right?

If all I've just shared seems like an awful lot to chew on, I can assure you it was. I didn't digest it very well myself. And after years of chronic stress, I experienced what ultimately appeared in the form of a cancerous tumor located directly inside my physical digestive system.

The years of hurt would eventually harden my heart. I spent a lot of time focusing on all that was going wrong in my own life and obsessing over the immense pressure of our many troubles, which then seemed to cause us to encounter further suffering and misery as a result. We magnified our problems, focusing on all the hurt, betrayal, and wrongdoings.

My broken heart and unimaginable stress manifested into physical suffering and illness. After years of chronic distress and dis-ease, it inevitably led to my disease. I hold no doubt that my cancer resulted from the stress experienced from our legal and financial struggles that wreaked havoc over my health.

Looking back, I believe my distress signal was sent out the day I abandoned my sinking ship. My call for help was answered. It arrived at the very last minute and in the most unexpected of forms. Cancer was the storm that saved me and blew me forward, carrying me to dry ground.

Without cancer, I never would have reached where I finally am today. I nearly drowned in the process and am lucky to have survived it, but I think it took sinking the whole ship for me to finally let go of everything else that I needed to release. I would never have done so willingly and without being forced. In my case, I needed to let go of wanting to have control over my happy ending. I needed to let go of the pain, bitterness, resentment, and fear I had accumulated and buried away deep inside my heart over the years. I needed to release all my suppressed emotions.

I HOPE THIS HELPS

If you're reading this, thinking, 'I wonder if I've got an overload of stress in my life,' I wholly recommend taking the Holmes-Rahe Life Stress Inventory Test. You can find many sites that allow you to take it online. It was one of the turning points for me in discovering just how much stress I had been putting myself under. And we all know just how poisonous stress can be to our bodies – you don't need me to remind you! Two psychiatrists developed the Holmes-Rahe Stress Test in the 1960s to establish at what point stress creates disease and illness in the body. Your result may bowl you over, but just taking the test will make you more aware of how you can better serve your body by keeping stress to a minimum – or at least as much as possible in today's age.

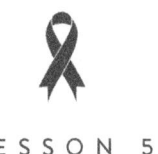

LESSON 5

MINDSET IS YOUR GREATEST MEDICINE

Early on in my journey, I instinctively knew that I must work my way through the fear, sadness, high stress, and grief that I experienced following my diagnosis. After digesting the news and finally arriving at the acceptance phase, I felt fully prepared to go in for the fight of my life. I had discovered a newfound confidence and was ready to face my future courageously.

I had an epiphany during a deep prayer one night that would help carry me through the remainder of my journey. It was an inner knowing from within my heart that I believe to be absolute truth. It became a mantra that I recited daily: *Mindset is the greatest form of medicine.*

I knew that I was going to need to become deliberate with my thoughts and feelings. I needed to make an effort to hold a higher perspective rather than give in to thoughts of defeat. I needed to listen to and trust the inner voice guiding me to develop a deeper connection to my body and get in touch with how I responded to everything around me.

I was ready to raise my level of awareness and chose my thoughts accordingly. I believed that cancer was happening for me, and for some higher reason. This prayer resulted in my gaining exceptional clarity about what I wanted to create and have unfold in my future.

It was as though this awful disease was part of my destiny and would allow me to become a greater version of myself. I had even prayed for explosive growth, blessings, and life transformation in the weeks leading up to my diagnosis. I wanted to become a healthier and happier person. Something that I had tried but failed at for years leading up to this fateful day.

Cancer certainly seemed like an unlikely solution to my problems and hardly an answered form of that bold prayer request, and yet, on that night in deep prayer, I had arrived at this moment of grace and utter peace where I somehow knew everything was going to be okay.

I knew this. I felt it with such certainty that I boldly proclaimed it mere days into this ordeal when first sharing about having cancer on my Facebook page.

I did so at a time when there was tremendous uncertainty around my future. I still had to discover the details of my prognosis and was waiting to learn what stage of cancer I had with no idea what survival rate was expected. Below is a section from that post.

Posted, 09:40 am, 08 December 2019

"This week, I was diagnosed with colon cancer.

My husband has been encouraging me to call others and share this information for moral support, but I haven't been able to bring myself to do so until today. Writing has always been therapeutic for me, so I choose to share the news here as the easiest way to get it all out.

Of course, I am sad... and have needed to allow myself time to grieve the changes. I wish I could be preparing for the holiday season and spending quality time with my family in place of all of this. A part of me lacks confidence around all the uncertainty for my future. I desperately wish I could wake up from what feels like the terrible nightmare I have been living over this last week.

I anticipate things will only get harder moving forward, but I know that mindset is the most powerful medicine.

This morning I am picking myself up, drying my tears, and digging deep to embrace the courage and faith I undoubtedly need to persevere through this.

Sometimes, life throws you unexpected interruptions and deep disappointments, but I genuinely believe there are good things found on the other side of suffering. I am ready to fight for my life and fully intend on coming out the other side of this struggle a stronger version of myself.

I will keep going. I will remain steadfast. I am prepared to put up with anything that comes my way. I will never lose sight of where I am heading.

I believe that God is good, even when life isn't good. This is how I will face this deep hurt, physical pain, and the inevitable suffering I expect to experience through treatment. Still, I will continue to run my race with oxygen filling my lungs, joy filling my heart, and peace filling my mind.

This is how you get through the harrowing twists and turns of life. This is how you make sense of all the things that don't make sense.

Cancer sucks, but I am strong and capable. I've walked difficult paths before, and I'll walk this one too while setting an example for others along the way.

God would never have allowed this without it serving some good. As hard as it is to make sense of here today, I believe this is happening for me.

I believe that someday sharing my story is going to be part of my life's purpose. My showing how an ordinary person like me is capable of doing the extraordinary. I will start by placing faith over my greatest fear and face cancer head-on."

It was a rather bold proclamation. Many marvel with me today over how those powerful words have since turned into my reality. It was as if, in my writing, I had somehow predicted my future, but with no way of knowing I could do any of it at the time.

I get goosebumps when I read that Facebook post. The morning I wrote that, it was as though something had taken over my thoughts, helping me find just the right words to express what my heart already knew, but that the rest of the world would have to wait to see.

I don't know how else to describe it, but I had a strange inner awareness that cancer was meant to be a part of my greater life story.

That same strange sensation has returned to me often as I write certain chapters of this book. I sometimes don't know where the thoughts I write originate, but I trust them wholeheartedly without needing to understand them.

It's true. I have accomplished much of what I set out to achieve and intended. The only thing that mattered on that fateful day when I first said the words aloud was that I genuinely believed it. I meant every single word, with every ounce of my being.

It didn't matter what the doctors' report would come to say. I didn't concern myself about what stage I would be diagnosed with or the scary numbers that my survival statistic would read. I only knew what I felt deep within my soul, and that my spirit was telling me that everything would work out exactly as it was meant to be.

I had a tremendous sense of peace with this thought. I believed that my story would one day come to serve a very important purpose, even if it had a sad ending in my not surviving.

Of course, I wanted to live. Now that I had finished grieving over the possibility of my death and the life I thought I was supposed to lead, I arrived upon a very important decision that day. Instead of focusing on all the reasons that I didn't want to die, I chose to transition my thoughts to the many, many reasons why I wanted to live.

What I find fascinating while typing this memory for you today is how, at the time, I didn't realize the tremendous power foreshadowing the thoughts in my head and feelings in my heart would come to hold over my future.

• • •

While I couldn't guarantee my outcome, what I did know was that my choosing to believe in what I wanted to happen made the likelihood of this occurring far more possible.

I have always been a believer that our thoughts create form. I'm a fan of Dr. Wayne W. Dyer and had recently finished reading two of his best-selling books, *There's a Spiritual Solution to Every Problem* and *Change Your Thoughts, Change Your Life*. One of his quotes spoke volumes to me: "Change the way you look at things and the things you look at change."

Dr. Wayne Dyer was a close friend of Dr. Deepak Chopra, another favorite author of mine. Both explain that the body has an infinite capacity for change and renewal. This topic has been written about by many, but I like their way of explaining this best. These authors share how quantum physics shows us how this all works and how we can use it to heal the body simply by using the mind. The more I read of their work, the more I wanted to explore.

I devoured every book I could find about quantum physics and came alive with the research and studies I found. In an article where scientists explain the world of quantum physics, I discovered that nothing is solid and everything is energy.[1] It sheds light on our world in ways that challenge the existing framework of accepted knowledge. What we perceive as our physical material world is not physical or material at all.

Science has shown us that every object is made up of tiny molecules. Molecules are made of tiny atoms. Atoms are made of tiny sub-atomic particles called neutrons, protons and electrons. If you were to observe the composition of an atom under a microscope, you would see small energy vortices called photons and quarks.

These are what make up the structure of an atom. Physical atoms are made up of vortices of vibrating energy that are constantly spinning, each one radiating its unique energy signature. (Yes, I like the science stuff!)

Quantum physics is the invisible world that makes up the solid objects from our environment. It is the study of matter and energy at the most fundamental level. The information started to sink in and make sense to me. If I was to observe myself and find out what I am at my most broken down core, I am a being of energy. I am always vibrating and radiating my unique energy signature.

I learned that if you focus on the structure of the magnified atom, what you would see is absolutely nothing. You would observe a physical void. You would conclude that the atom has no physical structure. In other words, that I (and you) have no physical structure. No physical things have a physical structure. Atoms are made of invisible energy, not matter.

Crazier yet, it turns out that at this tiniest subatomic level, the actual act of observing a particle changes the particle. Some argue that the way we observe these infinitely small building blocks is a determining factor in what they ultimately become. Mind-boggling, I know!

The key takeaway here is how, according to quantum theory, it's not such a huge stretch to imagine that the way we observe the world we live in affects that world. You could also say that the way we observe cancer and disease affects it. Your feelings about it and the perspective you hold over it result in your experience of it.

I decided from the very beginning I would apply quantum theory to my cancer. That's why I decided I ought to use mindset as my greatest form of medicine. My thoughts were as vital toward my recovery as the physical forms of my treatment plan, such as anti-cancer diet, surgery, and chemotherapy.

Changing the way you look at things is an extremely powerful tool. I knew I needed to become acutely aware of my thoughts and feelings to best position myself to heal. I understood that how I reacted, responded, and felt about everything that was happening to me held a direct connection to my odds of surviving it.

I understood the inextricable connection between the mind and the body. To be precise, I knew how the thoughts in my head and feelings from my heart ultimately translated to the physical experience I was having in my gut - or colon.

I also desperately wanted to experience a sense of inner peace and joy amid the health crisis. I wanted to balance my mental and emotional state for good and learn how to do so despite the chaos surrounding me.

To accomplish mastering my thoughts, I first wanted to better understand the complex science behind all my thoughts and feelings. I wanted to learn how to uncover, understand, and shift old patterns of thought behaviors that no longer served me.

I was introduced to a fascinating study of New Psychology Transformational NLP by Carl Buchheit, Ph.D., and Ellie Schamber, Ph.D., offering a new understanding of how the brain works.

Neuro-Linguistic Programming (NLP) is the study of the structure of human experience. It is a communication toolkit that provides the ability to discover, utilize, and change programmed thoughts and behaviors, assisting us in having new experiences in life that are more satisfying, fulfilling, and enjoyable.

Transformational NLP is a ground-breaking synthesis of psychology, Neuro-Linguistic Programming (NLP), and spirituality, bridging the domains of psychotherapy and coaching. While the practice looks like psychotherapy, it utilizes NLP and innovations drawn from quantum physics, psychology, and recent discoveries in neuroscience and systemic constellations. I read the book and can personally attest that it works. I am not the expert and suggest, if you are interested in learning more, that you visit their website at www.nlpmarin.com. While I am not an NLP expert myself, this study certainly opened the door for my willingness to learn more about how I could apply this to my catastrophic illness and work it favorably into my recovery efforts.

For the sake of mastering using mindset as the greatest form of medicine and wanting to get more in tune with the invisible power in my head, I wanted to dive deeper into understanding what science can tell us about thoughts.

Recent research into the human brain suggests that the average person will typically have more than 6,200 thoughts in a single day.[2]

That is an awful lot of thoughts. This number sounds accurate to me. I'll wager I may have more. I often wish I could turn the running commentary inside my head to "off."

My inner voice is a serious Chatty Cathy whose obnoxious conversation is annoying, even to me. I only wish I could find a mute button for my brain. It seems to amplify at night, reaching peak potential, usually right after I've crawled into bed and am ready to fall asleep.

"Did you remember to lock the garage door? I think so. Maybe I better go check. Wait! Did I buy those class supplies I volunteered to pick up for Taylor's science project? Tomorrow the kids have four sports practices at the same time in three different cities. That is going to be tough to juggle. Don't panic. You've got this, Supermom! Shoot, I forgot Sienna ran out of her favorite toothpaste. She's going to be so bummed I didn't grab more at the store earlier today. I really should write that down on the shopping list before I fall asleep and forget again tomorrow. Maybe I should try and go pee one more time before drifting off to sleep, so I don't have to get up again in an hour? Nope, way too cozy under these blankets. It's so warm and....

Darn it. I have another round of chemo tomorrow. How could I forget about that? I have cancer. That seriously sucks. Also, I really don't want to die. Why me? Stop it, Erin! You know better than to think like that. Focus and redirect your thoughts.

I want to live to grow old and have more time with my family. That's it. Now, try and visualize yourself ten years from now. You are at the twins' high school graduation. Go there. Feel it. See it. There it is! The kids look so cute in their caps and gowns, beaming with such pride. Awww, I'm not ready for them to grow up and move away to college. Wait, no more sad thoughts. Maybe I should fast forward another twenty years to when I am a grandma, still alive and kicking in my late 60's, spoiling my many grandchildren.

Search for it. Bingo! Look, there I am, all old and wrinkly, happy, and loving life. And there's Will. Hi, Honey! Look at us; we're grandparents. There are so many cute little ones running all around this place. Hey, how many grandkids do we have? Too many to count. I guess that's what happens when you have four kids of your own. That's gonna make for an expensive holiday shopping list.

Check it out! Will's still super cute as an old guy. I love him so much. How come I didn't age as gracefully as he did? This is my visualization, after all. Oh, no! There he is, over there asleep and snoring again. Wait a minute. Pretty sure that is him snoring in actual real life. So noisy. Great, now I'm never going to fall asleep."

All those thoughts above are what I'm capable of thinking in under five seconds flat. I'll bet closer to 10,000 thoughts flow through my crazy noggin in a single day.

Undoubtedly, every one of us is inundated with thoughts that appear to come and go freely, seemingly from some unknown source. The best I could do with all this wild information was to conclude that I needed to learn how to get incredibly deliberate with how I processed these thousands of thoughts and use them all to start working in my favor.

I decided to follow a three-step process. My unscientific way of practicing mindset as your greatest form of medicine was born out of all the reading I was doing and my urgent need to control the Chatty Cathy in my head. Step 1: Observe. Step 2: Contemplate. Step 3: Decide.

I carefully observed my thoughts and recognized all my feelings. I found that the key to practicing this was to be as calm as possible and avoid reacting or responding to whatever thoughts came into my mind, but rather simply become observant of them. The good, and also the bad. The thoughts that made me feel anxious, stressed, sad, and all the ones that made me feel happy and hopeful.

I contemplated all my thoughts objectively as best I could and started to recognize how some weren't serving me for good. I noticed how some caused me to feel panicked. How some raised my heart rate and even made my stomach turn. At the same time, other thoughts make me feel calm, relaxed, and safe.

I realized I always had a choice: I could either allow and accept every thought that popped into my mind or decide to choose another one. I became acutely aware of which thoughts I wanted to hold onto and which ones I opted to release because they weren't aligned with me.

I can always tell which thoughts are "off" based on how they make me feel. What settles as a good thought I can sense using my gut instinct. I pay close attention to how thoughts resonate within by gauging my body's response to them.

When I thought about my cancer, I focused on what I wanted, not necessarily what I saw—thoughts of hope over hopelessness. I transitioned from limited thinking to limitless thinking, where all things are possible. My full recovery and survival. My health and my future. I kept an open mind and never attached myself to what I was currently experiencing. I believed I was more powerful than cancer, not powerless to it.

I couldn't see how many of the things I thought about, daydreamed about, wished for, and wanted could work out at that time, especially when I was very sick. I only knew that the solution or how it could work didn't need to be identified.

I visualized often, and I saw myself as radiant, smiling, and in full health, living out the life of my dreams. If we can imagine it, why can't we achieve it? This change becomes possible when we understand how our brains work and are willing to make an effort to work with, and not against, ourselves. I did so during one of the most physically, mentally, and spiritually challenging times of my life.

I HOPE THIS HELPS

When it comes to survival, I, for one, was not willing to risk life and death by placing all my bets on just one team. I did my research and found ways to back up my medical team's work. I wanted to give myself the best chance, and I knew there could be ways I could help the process.

I concluded that it is best to treat the whole person rather than just treating the disease. My doctors were hard at work treating my cancer while I was busy completing the inner work I believe was behind the root cause.

Integrative healthcare is the term used for coordinating non-mainstream and mainstream elements to provide holistic treatment. This form of fighting disease bridges together the best of both worlds. In other words, you can use these complementary therapies together to build upon all else you are also doing in terms of your conventional medical care.

Putting all the power of your recovery into the hands of one team, whether that team is conventionally trained or holistically focused, is narrowing your odds, in my view. Why not use both? Why not pack your team with as many experts in as many areas as possible? That's why quantum physics and the power of mindset made such an initial impact on me. I was willing to believe in the expertise of others and boost my already strong treatment team. I suggest you do the same. find what works for you and create a power squad to help you heal.

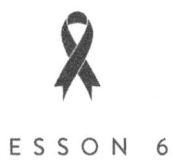

LESSON 6

YOU CAN CHOOSE TO BE HAPPY

Another secret commonly shared among cancer survivors is that they worked on increasing positive emotions. In my effort to get deliberate with my own thoughts and feelings to help me recover, I also decided I needed to increase feelings of joy and happiness over despair and defeat even when I felt anything but happy at the time.

I quickly found out in my research that when we feel happy, worry-free, and in flow, our physical bodies have a way of pumping powerful cancer-fighting immune responses throughout. Just as chronic stress has the effect of causing our bodies to create disease, increasing a positive emotional state does the exact opposite. It helps you heal.

In the book *Radical Remission*, author Kelly Turner states that making an intentional effort to experience more positive emotions is, in fact, a very important practice toward recovery, directly impacting your immune system. When you experience positive emotions, your brain releases a surge of healing hormones that flood your system. When I read this, I was overjoyed—and it had the instant mood-lifting effect that the research was talking about. These hormones, including serotonin, dopamine, endorphins, oxytocin, and relaxin, enter your bloodstream, helping the body by offering many healing advantages, such as:

- Helping your immune system increase both white and red blood cell count

- Helping your immune system fight cancer cells
- Clearing out infections
- Lowering blood pressure, heart rate, and cortisol levels (the bad stress hormone)
- Improving circulation
- Absorbing more nutrients from the digestive tract
- Oxygenating your cells through breathing. This is in contrast to not breathing, a common response when you are experiencing high stress or pain

I read clinical studies that correlated all the above physical reactions to positive thoughts and feelings, and it turns out laughter has one of the highest measurable health-inducing physical reactions. Laughing so hard that you cry is actually incredibly good for your health. How good is that to hear?!

Turner elaborates on how increasing positive emotions is beneficial for cancer patients. This has been shown to substantially improve the immune system's ability to remove cancer cells and recuperate from the damaging impact of certain cancer treatments' cellular damage, like that experienced from chemotherapy, for example.

So, with this knowledge in my back pocket, I sought every way possible to increase my happy hormones and give my immune system as much of a boost as possible, knowing it would get a shock once my body was subjected to chemotherapy.

I found that daily practices of gratitude, laughter, play, and creativity were all excellent ways for me to accomplish this. Music therapy is another powerful way to produce all the above-listed healing reactions without trying so hard on your part to create the feeling.

An easy way to practice increasing positive emotions is by using the words "I am." I recite a long list of "I am" statements in my daily mantras.

My favorites to recite are, "I am CANCER FREE," "I am BRAVE," "I am HAPPY," "I am A SURVIVOR."

Another time I used the power of "I am" was the morning of my cancer surgery. I posted a photo with my mother on the hospital gurney from the pre-op room, sharing my current status.

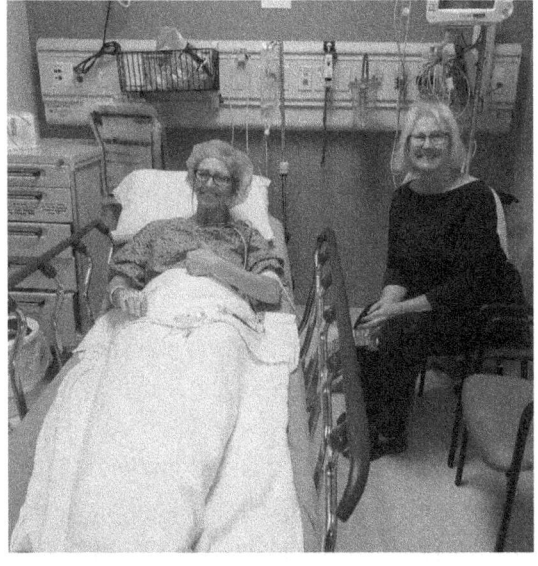

Dec 20, 2019 ·

I am STRONG.
I am CAPABLE.
I am COURAGEOUS.
I am LOVED.
I am HEALTHY.
I can DO THIS.
... See More

191   113 Comments 1 Share

And, indeed, I was, and I did.

• • •

These are empowering words, but I offer them with a word of caution: toxic positivity is a big no-no when working at increasing positive emotions. Please **DO NOT** fake it until you make it. I strongly advise against this popular advice.

Toxic positivity is the overgeneralization of a happy, optimistic state that results in the denial, minimization, and invalidation of the authentic human experience.

I discovered that during my seasons of stress and strife with our legal and financial struggles, I formed a bad habit of overusing positivity in my attempt to mask the pain, causing myself more harm, leading to the very suffering it was intended to diminish. Anything done in excess, like when positivity is used to silence the human experience, can become toxic.

I think it's safe to assume that none of us wants to be seen as a Debbie Downer, so when the choice is between a) be real and brutally honest, or b) pretend everything is awesome, we might be tempted to follow the latter.

Remember my conversation with the flustered "small problems" mom at school that one afternoon during my angry phase, when I had to bite my tongue from snapping a negative response at her? That was me taking the easy way out of the conversation.

I did so because, well, saying what I actually thought at the time would have been downright rude. Societal norms and etiquette prefer that we hide what we are thinking for the sake of others' comfort. In that instance, it was probably the right thing to do.

But bottling this kind of stuff up all the time eventually takes a toll. Maybe if I had just been honest when she had asked how I was doing, it would have been better and healthier.

Possibly, I should have said, "Thanks for asking. If I'm really being honest, I feel lousy. I was just diagnosed with cancer. I'm scared to death. I need a friend to just sit with me and listen. I need a hug. I need to let it all out and then have myself a long, hard cry."

I'm not actually suggesting you let in an absolute stranger you've only just met on all of your most private life dramatics - that's what therapists are paid for - but I now personally prefer to be a lot more real and whole during casual conversation, rather than always being "good" or "fine, thanks."

All smiles and acting as though all is well is a form of toxic positivity. The reality is that for many cancer patients, thinking and being positive is sometimes hard to do. I'd never suggested that anyone should try and force themselves to feel happy. That is unrealistic and also unhealthy advice.

Most of my friends describe me as an optimist, but the truth is I had become good at covering myself up and masking it over the years. I've personally battled with depression, anxiety, and all forms of negative emotions throughout much of my life. I also was always a people pleaser. I used to want everyone to like me. To understand me. To agree with me.

For a majority of my life, I hid my true opinions to fit in and for others to feel more comfortable being around me, and often at my own expense. It was exhausting.

No more. I have since found my voice and strive to speak my truth more often. In this book, I've already vulnerably aired some of my most personal thoughts, truest feelings, controversial opinions, and even a few of my most embarrassing memories and family secrets. I've become an open book, literally. No more faking it. I own it all now, the good and the bad.

Doing so has been freeing and feels friggin' fantastic. I encourage you to try and do the same as well. Get real. Be honest. Don't worry about whether or not others will accept or agree with how you think and feel. Of course, make an effort to be gracious toward others when doing so, but first and foremost, be authentic to yourself. In doing so, you will ultimately become a far happier (and healthier) person in the long run.

If others followed this advice, I'll bet we'd have far fewer people needing potent pills to ease their pain; way less stressed out, sad souls roaming around sick with depression. I have a family history of members who struggled or are struggling with anxiety and depression. This topic is very personal and something I am especially sensitive about when it comes to mental health.

• • •

During seasons of particular strife, like cancer treatment, increasing positive emotions could feel like a far-fetched goal. Should you find yourself struggling in this area, I strongly suggest seeking professional help from a therapist or psychiatrist and considering using medication if needed. For some, resources like these can be game-changing and incredibly helpful to increase positivity healthily.

Asking for help with your mental health takes courage, and I applaud those who do for their act of bravery—a valiant effort toward self-care. There are many free resources offered to cancer patients for this very reason; struggling with this is a very commonly shared experience.

I was fortunate to relieve my battles without the use of medication. I learned that I could overcome days when depression or anxiety seemed tough to manage by exercising, listening to music, watching a comedy, or doing activities that lift my spirits (like being around family or getting out in nature). These activities thankfully work wonders on my part.

As a cancer patient, you don't need to try to be positive all the time. Certainly, don't beat yourself up if you find yourself struggling. You should not fake it until you make it, nor should anyone expect you to be endlessly happy day in and day out.

The very thought of trying to always feel positive emotions can even lead to experiencing more strife. After discovering the damaging physical impact this has on my body in weakening my immune system, I sometimes get more anxious when I feel stressed or depressed. Give yourself a break and make an effort to gauge this.

To "just think happy thoughts" at a moment's notice is simply unrealistic for many. Sorry, Tinkerbell. You'll have to fly solo to Neverland, in that case.

The fact is, nobody is capable of feeling happy all the dang time, and I'm certainly not suggesting you should try this, either; especially when you need to feel and process the hard stuff. The last thing you should do is practice toxic positivity by avoiding, hiding, or running from the uncomfortable and icky feelings.

Consider that maybe an invisible guide in your head knows best. The one triggering your brain to think of the many things that mysteriously come to your mind is maybe doing so because you need to feel them. Even the bad ones. They are there for you to learn from.

Maybe your body has a natural ability to feed you these thoughts, offering you ample opportunities to practice mindfulness and getting deliberate with the 6,200 daily thoughts swirling inside of your head. To help you grow and eventually heal as you master observing, contemplating, and redirecting the ones you need to.

Fear, sadness, and pain all serve a purpose. As a cancer patient, it is virtually impossible to face the idea of death or to go through grueling treatment and not sometimes feel outright down and out.

It is natural to experience negative emotions. This is an authentic part of the human experience, one that can even be good for you providing you learn how to process them all for the betterment of your health.

Use mindset as your greatest form of medicine.

Just remember that all of your negative emotions have a shelf life. Be mindful over how long you allow yourself to experience them and recognize when they need to expire. Increasing positive emotions is proven to be good for your health. They say the best things in life are free. Happiness is one of those things because it is something everyone can access, even those who consider themselves a pessimist.

You are not happy because everything in your life is good, but because you decide to find the good in everything, including cancer. How you decide to view it will be key to helping you start to heal it. Cancer is not your crisis but your catalyst. One you can use to transform and heal your life for good.

Your mind holds the capacity to help you heal your body. A minor shift in vantage point, selecting a different thought, can carry quite the healing impact.

I went from feeling as though I was walking through the valley of the shadow of death to illuminating my mind to see how I could navigate my way through my darkest season.

I Hope This Helps

Mindset is your greatest medicine, so I am prescribing you three daily doses of happiness, starting with five-minute increments. Aim for a morning, midday, and evening joy ritual.

You will soon create a habit of happiness. Increase your daily intake until this practice becomes more of a natural pattern. I hope this chapter has opened your mind to the incredible power your thoughts hold to help you heal, bringing a whole new meaning to the pursuit of happiness.

I hope you now understand how stress and too much negative thinking can adversely damage your recovery. I shared this not to strike fear in you but to help you understand why you want to reduce stress and increase positive emotions. Doing so will lead to your having a higher quality of life and one that is both happier and healthier.

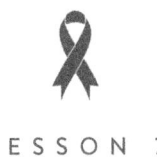

LESSON 7

RELEASE THE PRESSURE WHERE YOU CAN

Half a year before my diagnosis and during the days following my severe panic attack, we had decided it was time to regain some level of control over the stress-inducing factors we had been struggling with for so long.

Will and I both knew that this would require our making difficult family decisions and uncomfortable changes to better position ourselves to progress through and manage the legal and financial troubles that had been plaguing our family for years. That day on the floor of our bedroom, when we had hit our lowest point thus far, we arrived at making three very challenging life decisions for our family's future.

We were going to sell our beloved house and use any profit left over to pay off debt. After years of desperately grasping on to every possible attempt to avoid selling and saving our family home, we were finally tired of fighting to hold onto it any longer. Maybe it was never meant to be our forever dream home after all? We came to terms with that painful point despite it crushing both of our hearts. We focused on the silver lining of how this house had served us well for years as we welcomed our children and raised them in it. In those years the home had accrued equity. Equity that, once the house was sold, could be used to pay off debt as a means of helping us progress forward. There would be just enough to cover the overdue attorney's fees we owed and the future legal payments still likely needing to be covered. The home sale would provide enough cushion to cover our monthly expenses for a rental and our cost of living in the short term, without having to keep borrowing from family to help us survive. We were going to wipe the slate clean, once again, and start over entirely from scratch.

We were going to save up as much as we could for the future. To help us do so, we needed to cut back on our family expenses. That meant making some very tough choices, including one that directly impacted our kids. They were going to feel the impact that we had tried so hard to protect them from over the years. Losing their house would be painful enough, but we had also decided we needed to pull them out of their beloved school. We were taking away their home and now also their home away from home, and that decision hurt them deeply.

One of the largest expenses that we could save money on, however, was paying for tuition. This change would require a sacrifice on their part. It wasn't an easy choice for us as this had been the only school they had ever known since preschool. It was the other constant in their life apart from family and a place where they had love, moral support, and all their friendships.

Tuition had become a struggle over the years following the lawsuit, and we knew we couldn't afford to continue paying for school. Taylor was about to enter kindergarten and Liam was entering preschool. Tuition times four students wasn't a viable option, even with the financial aid we had received from the school. We needed to cut the cord entirely and save on this expense in our effort to free ourselves from debt. This news was not well received, and the kids pleaded with us not to make them leave their school, but we explained that we had no other option. Paired with the news that we were also planning to sell their home, this came as a brutal blow that upset the children. However, we knew that they are resilient, and with some time, this would eventually work itself out and get easier.

Losing our home and changing schools was a lot for everyone to come to terms with. While these decisions were necessary steps in the right direction, they left us heartbroken. We all suffered a tremendous sense of loss. The legal and financial burden was hard enough, but these changes were part of the growing ripple effect that we had to continue suffering. We decided that due to the many sacrifices we had made, we needed to allow ourselves one tiny win amid the disappointment—two giant steps forward and one little step back. We needed something to make it feel a bit more tolerable. We decided to book a last-minute getaway and focus on quality time spent together as a family. This vacation would take place at the end of summer, just before the kids started their new school year and right before we would list and sell our home in the fall.

This last decision was the one thing we did for ourselves. An act of self-care. It seemed counterproductive and a bit irresponsible considering our dire financial circumstances, but this would later prove to be one of the greatest decisions made for our future.

I happened across a last-minute, affordable monthly rental at our family's most favorite place on the entire planet, Costa Rica. It seemed almost too good to be true, perfectly timed, being available to rent just days following our conversation about our needing to take a family trip.

It seemed the stars had aligned. This trip was meant to be. We took the rental's availability as a sign to proceed. We took the plunge, bought six plane tickets that we couldn't afford, and rented our summer getaway that would take us far away from our many problems back at home.

The trip would prove to be a critical step in our healing process. It continued to pay off throughout the year following my cancer diagnosis. Ironically, it was booked to begin one week following my stress-induced breakdown after the horrific setback suffered from the lawsuit.

We nearly didn't leave for the trip because of how awful things had become from my meltdown and fragile state. Our family argued that it was justified even more for the sake of recovery, calm, and desperately needed respite. We needed this trip more than we realized. We somehow managed to pack our bags, drive to the airport, and board a flight to San Jose.

∙ ∙ ∙

A five-hour red-eye flight-with-four-kids later, we finally arrived. We decided to make a quick stop at the beach in Playa Sámara, to dip into the refreshing ocean and wake up from our jet lag. The sensation of the warm water instantly washed away all feelings of struggle and anguish that had been weighing so heavy on my heart. I completely forgot about everything left behind at home.

For a moment I was full of grace, my head was clear, and I felt nothing but a tremendous sense of peace and gratitude for the magnificence of that moment. Of course, our problems would all be waiting for us when we returned, but in that presence of the magic that Costa Rica offers, a tangible shift occurred inside, allowing us to feel safe for the first time in years.

This wasn't a typical family vacation. We had visited Costa Rica before and had already fallen deeply in love with this special place. We daydreamed about moving there one day with our family and spending an entire year living abroad, away from the chaos of life back at home. It was an escape fantasy, yet one we seriously pursued.

This trip was intended to be without bells or whistles because we didn't have the extra money to spare. We intended to avoid common tourist traps and excursions. We wanted to keep the cost to a minimum, eat at home and test out what it would be like to live like locals, often referred to as "Ticos" in Costa Rica.

We spent our days surfing the warm waters with the kids and visiting all our favorite beaches. It was a simple time engulfed in Mother Nature, and we stayed long enough to achieve perfection in the form of desperately needed relaxation.

That summer we temporarily managed to escape our pain and regained the strength we would come to rely on after we returned home. It was enough time for us to heal our hearts. For three and a half blissful weeks, we soothed our weary souls. We spent the trip letting go of all worry and embraced the Pura Vida lifestyle. This beautiful place allowed us to hit pause, come up for air, and fully rejuvenate our minds, bodies, and spirits.

I often visited Playa Sámara in my mind during my worst days of cancer, when I was too sick or weak to cope. I would close my eyes and take myself back to my happy place and the many beloved memories in it. I would visualize floating in the water alongside my family and instantly immerse myself in the cleansing and purifying ocean.

I could taste the salty water, hear the sound of the waves crashing ashore and watch as my children laughed and splashed around me. I would smell the sweet tropical flowers while the fresh sea air filled my lungs from the cool ocean breeze. I would feel the sand beneath my toes and walk myself deep enough into the surf to fully submerge my body, instantly dissolving my pain and troubles, time and time again.

This visualization was what got me through some of the absolute worst days when the discomfort from chemotherapy and cancer proved more than I could bear. This was the place I visited during my darkest hours. A place I prayed I would experience again should I be fortunate enough to survive.

Costa Rica is situated in one of the world's five blue zones. Blue zones are places on this planet where people live the longest, healthiest and happiest lives. In other words, they serve as model locations for living life the right way.

If you have ever had the fortune to visit this country, you will be familiar with the term "Pura Vida." Simply translated, it means "simple life" or "pure life." But in Costa Rica, it is more than just a saying—it is a way of life. There is a beautiful culture there. The people, the food. The tropical rainforest and pristine beaches. There is a lush environment with an ecosystem like no other place on the entire planet.

I truly believe that the beauty of the ocean can heal, and the beaches of Costa Rica are nothing short of a miraculous gift from Mother Nature. Ask those who have had the privilege to spend time in this magical country; they will tell you it is a truly special place.

That summer in Sámara provided our family with the desperately needed clarity and time to enjoy the simplest and best of life's pleasures. Costa Rica will forever be an important place for us. That summer trip left us inspired and filled with a renewed sense of hope. We were so thankful to have gone on that trip during the time we arguably needed it most.

We came to realize that our house back at home, the one we had been so intent on saving, was nothing more than a structure of beams. Our true home was wherever we were, even if that place was in a faraway country. Home is where the heart is, so they say. And as long as we were together, we were very much at home.

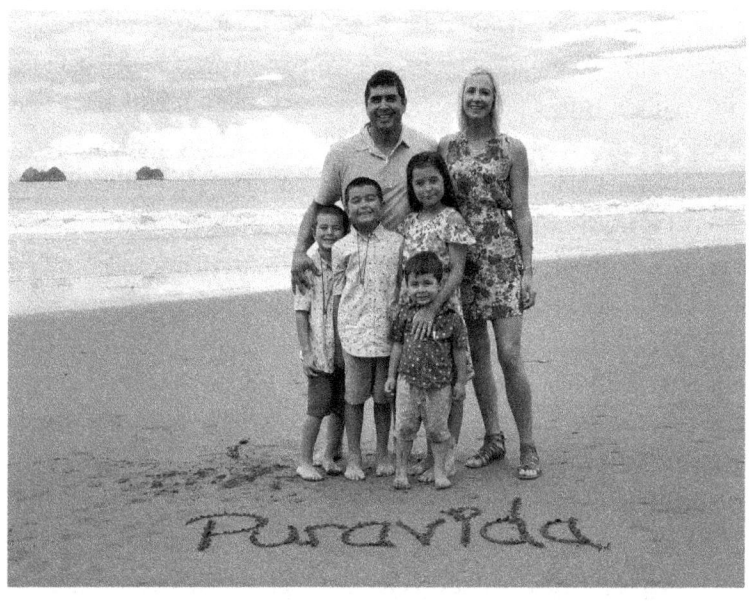

Pura Vida vibes from the Soto family in Costa Rica.

• • •

After that month, we arrived upon a significant fourth and final major family decision to help us change for good. Our time spent living as "Ticos" further solidified the choice that we knew would be best for our family's needs. It was the next step in figuring out how we would move forward in our life following all the hardships we had faced. That summer had helped us discover that, one day in the future,

Costa Rica very well could be our next home.

We had identified what school the kids would attend and figured out how we could live on a bare-bones budget for twelve months abroad with what we had left after selling the house and paying off legal fees. We would set aside all else we could save after paying off our debt with hopes that we could save up over the next year to prepare for the move. We thought of several ways to earn money, including projects we wanted to pursue while we lived there. After we returned home from our summer trip, we solidified this as our plan of action.

It was official. We were planning to move to Costa Rica in the summer of 2020. Looking back, nobody could have predicted catastrophic illness with cancer, or that a worldwide pandemic was mere months away, but after all that has transpired since, this dream is still just as much alive today as it was back in the summer of 2019. Arguably, more so now than ever before.

That September, we announced to friends and family our plans to move abroad next June. Saying it aloud meant we were fully committed and had to get to work following through on arranging everything required to make this pipe dream a reality.

Just before we left Costa Rica that summer, we had even found our dream house perfectly situated in the hills high above the tropical canopy overlooking a tranquil beach called Playa Carrillo. We named the property Sámara Sueños, which translates as "Sámara dreams."

We had been searching for a property with the help of local real estate agents who toured this particular home with us several times during our stay that summer. We felt an unusual connection to the home and were intent with our dream to purchase, renovate, and perhaps build upon the property sometime in the future.

It is a former family-owned home sitting in vacant disrepair for the last couple of decades, requiring a significant amount of fixing up to return to its former glory. The location has everything and more in terms of sheer perfection. Renovating properties is something Will and I still believe we can do successfully, and we would welcome the opportunity to tackle a challenge such as this should we ever be so fortunate.

The property has a large family home with a pool and plenty of flat space to build several guest homes. It is perched at the highest point on top of a mountain. It receives cool ocean breezes and has unobstructed panoramic views stretching from as far south as Santa Teresa north to Nosara. The sunsets here are majestic.

•••

After returning home, we were eager to share our enthusiasm for Costa Rica with anyone willing to listen. More importantly, we were on a mission to share something similar to our personal experience with those who might benefit from it most.

I had a wild idea to launch a nonprofit, envisioning how we could use the Sámara Sueños dream home for more than just our own family's year abroad, renovating it into a vacation rental income property open to anyone looking to renew and rest. We could share the place with others for the same purpose as it would serve our own needs.

The vision was to create a nonprofit organization with a mission of using the property to provide all-expense-paid vacations to families experiencing recent or ongoing hardship. It would also be used as a place to host group retreats for cancer fighters and survivors.

We would redefine what it means to travel and give back, offering vacations with a purpose to those who need them the most. I planned to use a portion of the profit earned from every paid rental we made on the vacation rental property to fund gift trips for others in need.

It was a crazy dream, but this property felt like a healing space that I couldn't shake my connection to after returning home. I formed a 501c3 called Sámara Sueños to get started on saving up and generating funds for both the house and travel expenses needed to cover those I hoped to provide vacations for in the future. I had even figured out ways to form partnerships with current vacation homeowners in Costa Rica, all willing to let me use their property for this purpose until we owned our own rental property.

When we eventually had our own house to rent out, I could fund even more charitable trips and cancer retreats without the expense of paying to rent others' places. And we could also finance the expense through charitable fundraisers and donations,

Keep in mind that when I had this grand idea and set up the nonprofit, I had zero connection personally to cancer. I was oblivious to the fact that I, myself, even had cancer this entire time.

A little ironic, don't you think? It still makes the hairs on the back of my neck stand up just thinking about it.

I really wanted this home to be a place for healing, not only for my own family to visit regularly and replenish, but for many others with whom we could proudly share. A place for more to find the same love and peace from it that we had.

As you can surmise, our original plans to move that summer were abruptly interrupted by my health crisis and Coronavirus, and we were forced to push this dream to the back burner.

While the opportunity to buy our Costa Rica dream home is not likely something we will see happen in our near future, I love holding onto the dream as something we will one day accomplish.

Dreams like that are well-worth chasing. I see the irony behind not knowing about my own disease and simultaneously forming the nonprofit as no mistake.

My personal cancer journey since has only further solidified my commitment to this dream. This is a future goal I hold close to my heart, no matter how long it takes for me to achieve it. This will be a home that my family and the many others fortunate enough to visit will enjoy for years to come.

If you are interested in donating to Sámara Sueños to support the future beach house property and sponsor sending deserving families experiencing recent or ongoing hardship from cancer on a trip to Costa Rica, please visit samarasuenos.org.

...

As planned, after returning home from our vacation, the kids started at their new school in the fall. We put our home up for sale by October, and it sold in less than a week. We asked to rent back the house through the holiday season in order to enjoy one final Christmas there before packing up and moving into our temporary six-month rental at the nearby apartment we had found.

The plan was to remain at the apartment through June while saving up for our move to Costa Rica that next summer. Escrow on our house closed the week just before that memorable Thanksgiving break.

A rule called Murphy's Law states, "If something can go wrong, it will, and usually at the worst possible time."

Something else happened for our family after my diagnosis that seems serendipitous when looking back. It deserves mention because you can see what happened as more than just bizarre luck; it is an integral part of this story worth mentioning.

When it rains, it pours. At the same time that my family's life was seemingly beginning to spiral out of control, my husband decided to leave his job as a managing partner of a large real estate office in South Orange County.

We were buried too deep in debt to keep living paycheck to paycheck, and my husband wanted to do something where he had more control over the income earned, something that could provide us with more consistency in pay and a much-needed sense of security. The timing felt right. He was ready for a fresh start and a new beginning.

It was early November of 2019 when he submitted his resignation, and two weeks later he worked his last day at the office, just in time for Thanksgiving break. Changing your job is always a risky move, and he had wanted to transition his career from real estate brokering over to lending.

Will struggled to land a position in lending after a background check showed our legal troubles had left us in debt, red flagging him as unfit to work in that space. He felt defeated and questioned that maybe he had made a terrible mistake in wanting to change his career path.

He wasn't originally interested when a listing agent position suddenly presented itself from a friend and former work colleague. Twenty years in the industry with a very successful track record of thousands of happy clients from residential sales meant he could always do the same thing he had been doing all the years before. But at first this did not appeal to him because it was going back onto the real estate side of business, not lending.

Will was adamant that the common pain points he struggled with from his former position needed to change. We had more than enough stress now to tackle following my new diagnosis, and he was concerned about adding more pressure to his overfull plate by continuing in the same position as before with a new employer.

My husband's friend insisted that Will come in for the interview before writing the company off. He explained how happy and less stressed he was after having made a move himself to work there.

There was no need to worry about where your next client would come from, as this real estate company's technical platform was the greatest in the nation, and clients come to them. As a large organization, their agents were treated as employees, which meant a steady and consistent salary and generous health benefits. That is a dreamy concept to most self-employed realtors who must cover their cost of medical insurance out of pocket.

Will agreed and went to the interview. The position he had applied for did not start for several more months, but they offered him a temporary job until the one he had been hired for could begin. He took the job, and then something unexpected and rather remarkable happened.

Another colleague, Erin, who also worked for the company, noticed Will's name as an onboarding employee of new incoming listing agents. Will and Erin had done business together many years before and were friends on social media. She knew about the new cancer ordeal our family was going through.

She took it upon herself to notify the CEO, informing him of our circumstances. He, in turn, ensured our health benefits began before my surgery, in order to help us cover the cost of my hospital stay. They wanted us to focus on my health and recovery rather than worry about paying our medical bills. We cried happy tears of joy, and to this day I still cannot believe what an answered prayer Will's new job and the company turned out to be for our family.

Will didn't have to do much in terms of "field" workload until after I had recovered from my operation. The first weeks entailed primarily office work. This better allowed time to take care of our family first until his new employee training officially began in January, after my December surgery. His company has a reputation for taking excellent care of its employees, and our family's new medical coverage was without question a blessing.

No longer worrying about how we would pay for my cancer treatment lifted a tremendous burden off our shoulders. I don't have to explain what a relief this was to us, especially given our financial circumstances.

Cancer is expensive. Those first few weeks of tests and treatment had already left us with $10,000 in medical expenses to cover out of pocket. Surgery was going to push us even into further debt. Every chemotherapy treatment, on average, costs $12,000, and we were frantic over how we were going to afford to keep me alive.

I see Will's timing in deciding to make a career change with a new company as being more than sheer coincidence; it seems an act of divine intervention. It happened as a result of the kindness of others who took it upon themselves to do us a desperately needed favor, one we hadn't asked for or expected, but will forever appreciate.

He still proudly works for this same company as a listing agent in South Orange County. Making his career move turned out to be one of his greatest professional decisions. He has never been happier with his work in all his 20+ years as a real estate broker.

The company also gifts its highest performers with annual

all-expense-paid trips. Out of all the wonderful places in the entire world, coincidentally, this year's trip is to—wait for it—Costa Rica.

With the lift of pandemic restrictions on travel, I may very well get to experience my dream of visiting Playa Sámara again, after all, post-cancer treatment.

Many say what a funny twist of fate and coincidence what happened to us was.

At first glance, we thought we were living Murphy's Law with anything and everything that could possibly go wrong, all happening at the most inopportune time. Looking back, I now see it all as a perfectly orchestrated series of events necessary to get us to exactly where we were meant to be.

I couldn't be better qualified to run a nonprofit serving families dealing with cancer. My husband's new job allowed him to focus on work while supporting our family and my health and offered us all the much-desired sense of security and peace of mind we had so desperately hoped for.

The home we sold and moved out from resulted in our now setting down new roots in another home in which we couldn't be happier. Arguably, it's a better one than the beloved one we lost. I would never have guessed any of this could be possible had you asked me this same time last year. What a difference a year can make in life.

Our life seemed hopeless and in a state of absolute disrepair, but we never gave up hope or succumbed to defeat. We kept our sights set on victory and placed all our faith over fear in every aspect of life.

In the end, despite not seeing how we could pull through it all, we managed to do just that. We not only survived, but we grew and thrived through it. We have since come out on the other side far better off than we were going into it.

I have come to know that divine interventions occur far more frequently than realized. Things have a way of working out, often when you least expect it and in a manner you never could have envisioned on your own.

Have you ever noticed this in your own life? How, out of the many big and little decisions made each day, there seems to be some perfectly orchestrated plan to it all? You are constantly receiving signs from above when stumbling across sudden twists of fate. If you are receptive to recognizing these when they occur in your own life, I find they tend to happen even more. Trusting the universe, even when it seems the outcome may be more than dismal, is the ticket to freedom.

I guess my family was long overdue for a lucky break, but I see what happened to us as something more than sheer luck. I recognize that these crazy coincidences, those I've shared and the many others that I have not, are answered prayers. The year of my cancer crisis served an important purpose, creating significant life transformation for our family. I now have a long list of unusual events I have difficulty explaining to others. There were setbacks that turned out to be setups for something better. Doors closed that later opened new ones offering bigger and better opportunities.

I Hope This Helps

They say life always is happening for you, not to you. I believe this to be true, especially in my own experience. I've experienced one too many stories of defeat that turned out to be those of victory.

Have you ever asked a question during prayer or deep thought and received an answer that came in the most unusual form? A conversation with a stranger later that day, lyrics to a song, a scene on the news at the very moment you happen to turn on the television, words that appear to jump off the page as though they were intended for you alone?

As you continue throughout this book, I encourage you to start looking for instances like this that occur in your own life. Consider that whatever problem you are currently facing could offer more than what it appears to at first sight. Cancer included.

These moments are powerful proof. Experiences that offer you hope when you need it most. I challenge you to be more open-minded in recognizing coincidental synchronicities in your own life. Especially during life crises and trauma, as these tend to be powerful moments when most miracles occur.

I know through personal experience that when you are tuned in expectantly and search for and are receptive to signs, these things have a way of finding you. Call it what you will. Coincidence, fate, an answered prayer, or a wink from the universe. It is all here to remind you that there are always greater forces at play—should you choose to see life for what it truly is.

PART III

How to Heal the Body

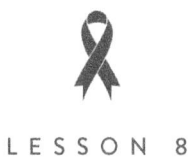

LESSON 8

KNOW WHAT YOU'RE WALKING INTO

Things moved very quickly after my cancer diagnosis. Time wasn't on my side.

Dr. Dalal had informed me during Friday's phone call that she had already scheduled an appointment for me with a surgeon, Dr. Sanders, come Monday morning.

Looking back, I can now see that, even before the biopsy results came in for the colonoscopy she'd performed on Tuesday, Dr. Dalal suspected I would likely be requiring lifesaving surgery. I am so appreciative of her quick response and for her helping with continued momentum to get me into the next set of healing hands.

I asked that both Will and my mother accompany me to this next appointment. The three of us were pretty much nervous wrecks as we anxiously waited for Dr. Sanders to arrive. My mom tried to look at ease, but she was tapping her shoe on the floor a thousand beats a second, like she was playing the drums. Will was rubbing the stubble on his chin with his fingers. I was twirling my hair in my fingers with one hand while biting my nails off the other, sitting on the exam table in my hospital gown, ready to meet my cancer fate.

We were all in the tiny exam room together, waiting in dreaded silence for what was to come. There was a knock on the door and then in walked a pistol of a surgeon who carried herself with a powerful presence. I cannot tell you what a relief it was to meet Dr. Sanders for the first time.

She had the exact kind of confidence you want to see when meeting with the surgeon expected to operate on you for cancer. Dr. Sanders has reddish-brown hair and striking green eyes, and she entered the room with her head held high and a slight smile on her face.

"Hello, Erin. Nice to meet you. I'm Dr. Sanders. I'm going to be your surgeon." She reached out her hand to firmly shake mine, making direct eye contact. "I'm here today to talk about what we need to do to save your life!"

I exhaled a giant sigh of relief. I knew instantly I liked her a lot. She got right to the point, reminding me how cancer is a word, not a sentence. It was the first time since receiving my diagnosis that someone seemed confident this was nothing but a bump in the road that I was capable of tackling.

It was at that moment I stopped wondering about whether I was dying and instead started thinking about how I was going to survive. It was when I decided to stop viewing my cancer as a death sentence and, rather, chose to see the experience as a life sentence for healing. It was now time to fight and push myself toward everything needed in order to live. Time to stop waiting and pass go. That appointment, when first meeting Dr. Sanders, was incredibly refreshing. Her belief in my ability to live beyond my cancer immediately put all of us at ease.

It is said that a good physician treats the disease while the great physician treats the patient who has the disease. Dr. Sander's reassuring first words gave me the strength to push through my fear and prepared me to move forward and learn more about my upcoming operation.

My confidence only grew as we learned how highly qualified she was. She shared information about her many years of experience performing this same procedure successfully many times before. She shared positive stories of patients who have since fully recovered and been able to get back to life cancer-free. Hearing her speak as though this was precisely what she expected to also accomplish in my own case was a comfort. She was a care partner I needed on my team.

Dr. Sanders walked over to a poster on the wall that displayed the inner workings and anatomy of the large intestine.

"I've just finished reviewing your charts and, from the looks of your CT scan, your tumor is located right here." She placed her finger on the chart, pinpointing the location of my cancer. "This area is called your sigmoid colon and is located just beneath your descending colon and above your rectum. Your mass is located about 6 inches up inside of your colon, and we are going to remove it."

She explained that her plan was to perform what is called a hemicolectomy. That is the medical term for surgery for colon cancer. It involves removing the part of the colon where the cancer occurs, as well as a small amount of normal colon tissue a few inches on either side of the tumor. So, for me, about six inches of colon, give or take. Lastly, the nearby lymph nodes are also removed. The plan was to cut my colon apart and carefully resect it back together, hopefully in working order.

"In other words, Erin, your pipes are clogged," she said. "My job is to perform some basic plumbing."

For the first time since hearing the big bad C-word first uttered days before, both my mom, my husband, and I were now all relaxing a bit. Dr. Sanders has a way of delivering serious news and information in just the right tone. She could tell upon entering that room, from the looks of desperation on our faces, that we were scared to death. Somehow, within minutes, she had every one of us feeling hopeful.

She went on to explain how this surgery is required when colon cancer has grown beyond the colon wall, and that we wouldn't know the extent of the cancer's spread until after surgery. The procedure itself would be done laparoscopically through two incisions in the abdomen, using long, narrow instruments inserted through the small incisions. The instruments contain a video camera to allow Dr. Sanders to see inside the body.

Depending on how things appeared after she got working on my insides, there was always the possibility that she may need to cut open more of my abdomen. She hoped to avoid this for future bikini shots come summertime; but, with saving my life as priority number one, she explained the possibility that my vanity may, if necessary, have to be brushed aside. She promised to try to keep the scars as minimal as possible, though. Her end goal was to perform a safe and effective operation with a healthy outcome, and she assured us all that she would do whatever was necessary to accomplish that.

I told her that if she needed to turn me into a walking Frankenstein, by all means, go for it. I did appreciate her plan to make an effort to leave less of a mess behind in the name of vanity, but my goal was to live to see my kids grow up. That's really all I cared about.

I teared up explaining how much I loved my family and practically pleaded with her not to let me die from this disease and operation. We had a little moment together, and she then reassured me everything was going to be alright. She could tell I was tough and encouraged me to believe in myself and her as my surgeon. Together, we were going to get through this.

My tumor was partially blocking my colon. She went on to explain that she hoped to avoid the need for a colostomy bag during the operation. Sometimes this procedure, called an ileostomy, requires a temporary bag while a colon connection heals. Surgeons always try to reconnect the colon back together again as best they can. Worst case scenario, she warned that I might wake up with an external poop bag. Although only a slight possibility, I needed to be prepared for this. Thankfully, this was avoided during my procedure, but I did worry about what that would have been like.

Dr. Sanders told me that my CT scan had shown a few lymph nodes just outside the colon wall that she was concerned about. During my operation, she would perform a lymphadenectomy, which involves removing and testing lymph nodes for cancer.

"This is how cancer spreads," she said. "In your case, the scan showed that your cancer does not appear to have spread to any of your surrounding organs yet. This is very promising news; when that happens, it means patients will need to continue further cancer treatment following surgery. That is what we hope you will not require. However, if cancer is detected in your lymph nodes, you will be considered to be at an advanced stage and you will then go on to meet with an oncologist to discuss ongoing cancer treatment options."

•••

So, for now, the plan was to get me into surgery and hope for the best. That next part of ongoing cancer treatment is not her area of expertise. Her goal was to remove the tumor in time to hope we might avoid that next phase of cancer treatment, which would likely involve chemotherapy or, as she lovingly referred to it, "the poison."

She went on to explain that "the poison" was basically a potent punch, a chemotherapy cocktail that would wipe out my cancer cells. It would also damage my healthy cells while slowly deteriorating my overall health. An oncologist administers this very carefully to only kill the cancer cells, and hopefully not you, during the process. It is a highly effective form of cancer treatment, but one we really hoped to avoid, if we are so lucky, because that carries on the cancer journey due to an outcome none of us are going for.

On the bright side, colorectal cancer has the highest survival rate when caught early. "Early" meaning Stage 1 or Stage 2, where the cancer cells have not breached the wall of the colon and spread to lymph nodes or surrounding tissue and organs. If they remain inside the wall, surgery alone will be curative. Remove them, recover, and move on with your life with no evidence of disease.

While we would remain cautiously optimistic in hoping for the best, we, unfortunately, wouldn't know more until following my operation. So, for now, our game plan was to prepare for surgery as soon as possible.

Dr. Sanders acknowledged this procedure was going to be anything but simple. It all was far more complicated than she was making it appear in conversation, but that was for her to worry about as my surgeon. The point was, I was in excellent hands. She does this often and quite well. The operation itself could take up to six to eight hours and would require four to six days to recover in the hospital after that. We shook hands again, and I left that appointment feeling like I was ready to crush cancer, eager to get under the knife that would cut out my tumor and hoping to leave this nightmare behind.

I had just met my surgeon-soulmate. Her track record was impressive, and I instinctively felt that she was the right person to perform my operation. I trusted her with my guts. Thankfully, it would turn out to be an excellent decision.

•••

My surgery was scheduled for Friday, December 20, precisely two weeks after I had been formally diagnosed by Dr. Dalal.

As I shared a bit before, this whole cancer news kind of put a downer on what was supposed to have been a joy-filled holiday season. Our family did very little to prepare for Christmas. Between packing to move out of the house we had "rented back" through the end of December, my now many frequent medical appointments, and how quickly everything seemed to be proceeding, we were just trying to keep going, coming up for some air when needed along the way.

Those two weeks flew by. On the day of my twins' eleventh birthday, December 18th, all the kids began their winter break from school. My dad and stepmom arrived just in time for us to attempt a celebration for the twins by taking everyone out for a birthday dinner at their favorite restaurant.

We put forth a valiant effort to be festive but weren't very convincing. Neither of my twins bought into our facade, nor did they have their usual birthday spirit. They understood the severity of the possible outcome of my upcoming surgery. My being sick seemed to steal their birthday magic and the spirit of the holidays we typically enjoy.

I don't think either of the twins expected anything big to happen for that year's birthday celebration, either, but they seemed appreciative of our attempt to make sure they enjoyed a slice of cake that night.

They cracked a few forced smiles for everyone at the dinner table, but I could tell what they were really feeling was uneasy.

The high emotions from that night still hurt. I sometimes wish I could do over their 11th birthday. That year we were just grateful to have our family all together, and we intended to make the most of the next 36 hours prior to my operation.

There was a possibility I wasn't going to be discharged to make it home in time for Christmas. My parents' job was to help Will with the kids during my hospital stay and to try to help them experience some remnant of what a normal Christmas should feel like, regardless of what was to happen with me at the hospital.

The next day my stepmom baked her delicious holiday fudge and cookies for the kids to decorate and eat. The baking filled the house with sweet smells while we all listened to Christmas music. No solid food for me; I tried to merrily choke down my third gallon of colon cleansing juice as my pre-op preparatory procedure required that I again starve myself on clear liquids and thoroughly clean out my pipes for Dr. Sanders' unclog.

That evening before surgery I had a difficult time falling asleep. I was anxious over the risk of the operation and the unknown outcome of my cancer status that this carried with it. It all had me feeling too jittery to rest. Everyone had gone to sleep, and Will and I were in our bed with Liam cuddling between us. Will had already drifted off, and Liam was holding onto me tightly like a little koala bear, attached snugly with his tiny arms and legs wrapped around my sides. We were nose to nose on the pillow, and his little baby breath was gently hitting my cheeks. I marveled at how innocent he seemed.

I wondered what the next few days were going to be like for Liam and everyone else in the house with my being away in the hospital. I thought about how worried my kids had been over the last two weeks and was overwhelmed with a sense of helplessness, wanting nothing more but to shield them from going through all of this and possibly forever ruining their memory of Christmas.

I gently kissed Liam's head and pulled him in close while I started to cry into the pillow we shared. My shoulders were bobbing up and down, and my throat ached as I tried to muffle the sound to not awaken Liam or Will. As I cried there feeling incredibly somber and sorry, I recalled how just a few weeks prior I had done another strange thing that now came to my mind. I began to wonder if possibly I had somehow brought this all on myself and my family.

• • •

A couple of weeks before my diagnosis, on the emotionally heavy day when we had closed escrow officially selling our house, I experienced another one of the rather peculiar coincidental crazy things. I went for a long run that morning to enjoy the neighborhood I had come to love so much over the years. I was trying to soak it all in before the move, and while jogging along my favorite part of the path I found myself lost in the form of prayer. I prayed for something that now came back to me, striking my heart like stone.

I often listen to audible books, podcasts, or motivational messages from some of my favorite inspirational thought leaders and authors while I run. That day, I was listening to a famous minister who was talking about how, when we go through a hard time in life or feel like we are stuck, we can become slaves to our unfortunate predicaments. It is during these times that we begin to lose hope and feel like there is no way out. It also is when we feel most lost and vulnerable that miracles are ripe to occur. The truth is that God wants to bless you; not just offer you a way out of your worst situations but help you to rise above and grow beyond them.

The minister then shared a prayer that I had repeated out loud. I stopped my run and prayed with every part of my soul. I fell to my knees alone in a field of grass and autumn leaves under the misty morning sky. I raised my head up and held out my hands, asking that God do great things through me. That God might use me and my struggles to show my true strength and allow me to serve as an example and instrument of peace. I prayed for explosive blessings and life transformation. I asked God to do something extraordinary in my life that would serve as a message of hope for others.

I meant it all when I said it, too. I held my hands together and then placed them onto the ground. I then sat in the field with my eyes looking up at the cloudy sky for a long while, sending that bold request for life intervention right on up and out into the universe. At that time, I was still thinking about the house sale and legal struggles. I thought I was praying to heal the hurt in my heart from feeling that others had cheated, harmed, and betrayed us deeply.

That evening in bed, now weeks later, I was dwelling over how foolish I had been in that fearless prayer. Then I was filled with a sense of anger as I recalled all I had asked for. Then back to feeling incredibly afraid for my surgery that next morning. My thoughts were now taunting and plaguing, keeping me from sleep.

I spoke aloud, directly to God, with my tear-stricken face in my pillow. "How could you do this? That was not what I meant when I prayed for that. I don't understand this. Cancer. Why did it have to be with cancer? I can't do this. I'm not ready to die. I'm so scared. Please. I don't want any part in this. Just take it all back. I didn't mean it. Make this all go away. I'm so sorry. Maybe I wasn't grateful enough for what I had before. I see that now. My problems were small compared to what I have now. Please, help me. Heal me."

I wept uncontrollably while begging for mercy. I pleaded for my life. I swore to God that if I were allowed to live through this, I would change my life for good. If only God would let me.

In the same moment when I was starting to question my faith, I had the most remarkable experience and sensation. In an instant, all the pain, agony, fear, distress, and rage suddenly lifted. I had been grief-stricken and heartbroken one second, and in the next, I felt a sensation overcome my body that felt warm and very safe and so comforting.

There was a strong presence that took over everything I had just been experiencing moments before. It felt like liquid love was washing through me. Something was breathing life into me. The heaviness in my heart was replaced with a lightness. There was such an intense feeling of pure love. I stopped caring about everything and just leaned into this feeling. It felt like a deep sense of inner knowing. It felt familiar, and it felt so right.

Was I dreaming? I still felt alert and awake and fully understood I had cancer, with surgery only hours away. But I no longer cared about the risks or even about my own death. No, I was not asleep, but I was terrified to move or open my eyes in fear that whatever omnipresence was surrounding me might disappear if I did. It was dark in my room and my eyes were closed shut, but I felt surrounded by light. I allowed whatever this was to soothe me. I asked aloud for this to please stay and help me fall asleep.

I was consumed with a strange sense of utter bliss and elation. My body no longer hurt from hunger, pains, and sickness. I no longer felt frightened in the slightest. I only had a tremendous sense of comfort and unconditional love. This moment was like nothing I had ever felt before, and it is hard to describe anything feeling close to this. This sensation was real and so intense. I realized I was still crying, but now only happy tears of extreme love and joy. I was now smiling on the pillow, and I continued to embrace Liam while I relaxed into this remarkable experience.

I was at more peace during those few minutes than in all my life before. I again thought to myself, as I had only weeks before in the middle of the night on Thanksgiving Eve, "Maybe this is what it actually feels like to die. Maybe this time, though, I really *am* dying!" The strange part is that now that thought in no way bothered or upset me. I was experiencing such a powerful sense of pure love that I can honestly say I would have been perfectly okay to die right then and there at that very moment. I didn't actually want to die, but in that moment I wouldn't have minded whatsoever if I had, as I never wanted to leave this intense sensation. I was at complete peace. I didn't want whatever this feeling was to stop. I also knew that I was very much still alive and that I was still lying in my bed. I knew this with certainty. So, I lay very still and calm, allowing whatever this was to blanket me from head to toe in pure grace.

I peacefully drifted off to sleep and, when I woke up the next morning, I was still carrying the sense of calm from the night before inside of me. I went to the hospital for my surgery.

•••

On the day of my operation, we left the house at 4:30 in the morning, deciding that with all we had ahead of ourselves, it was best to kiss the kids goodbye while they were still asleep and in bed. We wanted to keep it less emotional for everyone and also it would be easier to get out the door quickly.

I could still feel the strong sensation of peace within and was in bright spirits and ready for the operation. My mom, my stepdad, and Will accompanied me to the hospital that morning while my dad and stepmom stayed at home to care for the kids.

I should have been nervous, but I was unusually calm. Noticeably so, as even the admitting nurses, my surgeon, and Will asked me how I was so at ease. They admitted me into pre-op and when the time came for another cocktail from the anesthesiologist, I easily fell asleep without worry. I awakened eight hours later in the recovery room, with Will holding my hand at my bedside.

"You did it," Will whispered into my ear. "It is done. You are going to be okay. The surgery was a success and couldn't have gone any better. Now you just need to rest and relax so that we can bring you home as quickly as possible."

I was told to focus on my recovery in the hospital while we awaited the results. My family visited daily and kept me close company; we watched holiday movies and cuddled together in my hospital bed. Sienna had gifted me with a beautiful soft blue blanket covered with

Costa Rican sloths. We snuggled into it. We were all happy.

On the fourth day of my hospital stay, Dr. Sanders came in during her morning rounds to confirm I was going to be discharged that afternoon, in time to be home for Christmas Eve. I was so ecstatic to make it home for the holidays with my family. I thanked her profusely. Then her demeanor changed, and she sat down in the chair beside my bed.

"I am so happy to be able to share the good news for your discharge. But I am afraid I am here because I have some sad news that I need to share with you as well. The results from your surgery have come back. It confirmed that cancer was detected in two of the 24 lymph nodes I had tested after removal during your operation. I am afraid surgery was really only the beginning, Erin. I am so sorry. I know many patients who have gone through this before you and have fully recovered, so please do not ever lose hope. The surgery was a success, and you can still beat cancer through treatment."

It was difficult news to hear, on Christmas Eve no less, but I was ready to go home and still try to enjoy Christmas. I understood that everything I'd been through over the last few weeks, and the surgery I was now recovering from, barely scratched the surface of what was to come next in my fight with cancer.

I was discharged home to enjoy the holiday week with my family. An appointment had been set up for me to meet with an oncologist the first week after the new year in January of 2020. What a year 2020 would turn out to be!

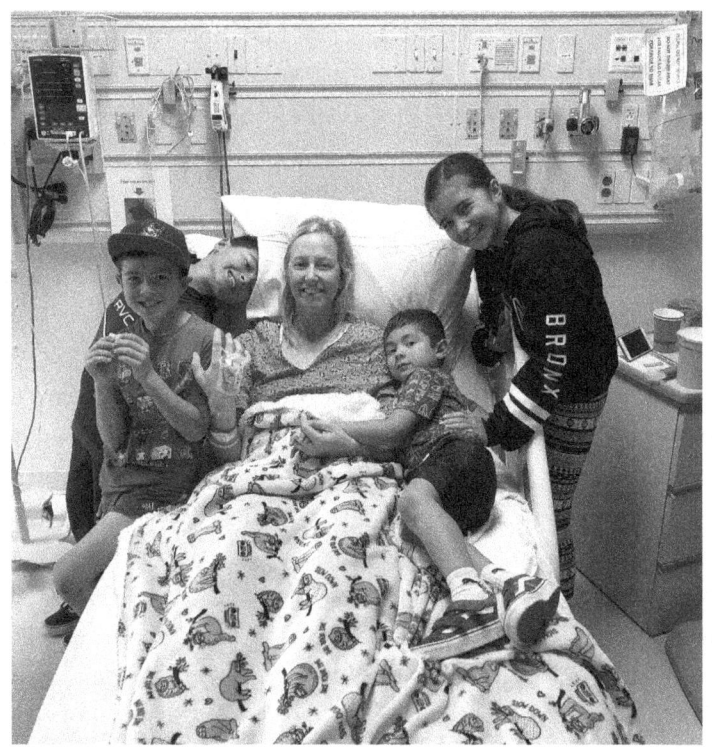

A Christmas wish come true. Discharged and heading home for the holiday.

• • •

We enjoyed Christmas and the New Year as best we could. I took a couple of weeks to recover from the surgery and gain back strength while we moved out of our house and into the apartment. I was scheduled to meet with my oncologist the first week of January while Will was away training for his new job in Atlanta.

My dad was still visiting, and he and my mom took me to the appointment while my Aunt Lynne, who had come from Arizona to help, was in charge of the kids. Dr. Parker is quiet-natured. He is close to my age with black hair, kind eyes, and a comforting smile. He is an excellent listener and is always very careful and selective with his choice of words.

He informed us of everything there was to know about chemotherapy, taking all the time we needed to answer our many questions. He explained that I was formally diagnosed with Stage 3 colon cancer—an advanced form.

"That sounds serious," I said. "How many people survive Stage 3 colon cancer?" I asked.

"I hate to answer this question because the reality is that no two patients are ever the same. While your treatment will be the same as for many other patients with your disease, outcomes vary," Dr. Parker said.

He explained there would be no way of knowing exactly how my body would respond to the treatment. Sharing the stage of my cancer, my projected survival rate, and the medical report might even cause unnecessary concern; however, he was willing to share the details if I wished.

"I first want to assure you that, despite what the report reads, we are going to do our very best to save your life. You are 37 years old, and aside from having cancer you appear to be strong and in excellent health," Dr. Parker said. "Sadly, I still have no way to guarantee results for any of my patients from this treatment. I also caution against giving too much weight to your survival statistic. You are not your medical report. I have seen patients do remarkable things against the odds."

He went on to add that my strength and age could be considered an advantage in being able to withstand the grueling impact of the cancer treatment he was prescribing, over other patients with health conditions similar to that of my own.

I told Dr. Parker that I am a distance runner, a fighter, and I regularly push the limits of the average person by testing myself. In fact, I explained he should not consider me his usual patient. "I welcome challenge, although I'd have preferred to skip on this run with cancer." I told him that I even planned to continue to run throughout my cancer treatment. He loved my spirit and respected my wishes.

"I promise I won't allow the scary statistic or this medical report to define me. I am stronger than my chance of death and this disease. I do still want to know what my overall risk is, though. I believe that my survival will ultimately be up to me," I said. "My mindset is what matters most. That, paired with all else that I am doing in addition to chemotherapy, really counts. I can assure you that in the month since being diagnosed, I have already radically changed much of my lifestyle to set myself up for success. I am working with you for my conventional treatment but going the full distance with integrative health practices to further improve my odds. That said, I'd still like to know what these odds are. I promise it won't deter me. I'm more determined to live than I am afraid to die."

...

Dr. Parker explained that in Stage 3 colon cancer the tumor has spread beyond the lining of the colon and to nearby lymph nodes. In my case, two of the 24 lymph nodes tested positive. Although the lymph nodes contained cancer cells, the disease had not yet spread to distant organs.

With treatment, many Stage 3 colon cancers can be placed into remission, meaning that the signs and symptoms of cancer will disappear, in some cases forever. For others, remission may be partial, and the treatment is used to slow disease progression, improve a person's prognosis, and increase the length of survival.

With improved therapies and treatment protocols, people with Stage 3 colon cancer are now living longer than ever.

There are also different types of colon cancer, some of which are common, like mine. I had what is called adenocarcinoma.

The biopsies of my lymph nodes and my tumor had been sent to a pathologist. That is someone who specializes in the causes and effects of the disease. The pathologist provided the results by which my cancer is characterized, staged, and graded. In other words, a pathologist provides you with your dreaded prognosis. Staging and grading are processes by which the extent and severity of the cancer are determined. These tests help direct the course of cancer treatment as well as predict the likely outcome of your survival.

I already had begun cancer treatment with my surgery. Stage 3 colon cancer is typically treated with surgical resection. Dr. Sanders had removed the affected portion of my colon. My partial colectomy was accompanied by the lymphadenectomy in which 24 nearby lymph nodes were removed.

Generally, a lymphadenectomy—a.k.a. lymph node dissection—is considered adequate when at least 12 lymph nodes are removed. The number of lymph nodes removed is based on a variety of factors, including the extent of the resection, the location and grade of the tumor, and finally, the age of the patient. The more nodes they can remove and test will offer better insight into your treatment and accurate staging and grading.

Most Stage 3 colon cancer patients will receive a recommendation of surgery, colostomy, chemotherapy, and possibly radiation.

•••

Chemotherapy is typically used in adjuvant therapy, meaning that it is delivered following surgery to clear any remaining cancer cells from the body. Dr. Parker explained that my lymph nodes are like a highway system to my entire body. Colon cancer that spreads to your lymph nodes often spreads to the liver and/or lungs. My liver was already enlarged when viewed in my cancer scan but, so far, no cancer was detected. Our goal was to wipe out any cells in this highway system that were en route to spreading to other parts of my body. We needed to get moving on treatment quickly.

My specific chemo cocktail was considered very potent. The chemo regimen they were going to give me was true to Dr. Sanders' description, like a toxic kick of poison. The goal was to knock out any remnants of cancer cells still possibly existing within my lymphatic system. They were going to give me the strongest and fiercest regimen my body could withstand.

I knew I needed to view chemo not as "poison" that could harm me, but powerful poison that I was strong enough to conquer while it worked *with me,* not against me, obliterating those pesky cancer cells on contact.

Dr. Parker then explained that, with this chemotherapy regimen, it is quite common for many patients to not finish all 12 rounds; however, the goal was to have as many sessions as my body could tolerate, increasing my odds of survival. Our hope was that I could handle as many rounds as possible, with each improving my odds of annihilating any lasting cancer cells so that they never come back.

While some patients can only withstand six to eight rounds, we would closely monitor and see how many I could handle working toward twelve. But do not fret if we needed to adjust my treatment or end early if my body reached a point where it was no longer safe to continue.

"Think of this as your greatest run yet, Erin," Dr. Parker said. "Remember that this is not a sprint. It is a marathon. It will be long and arduous and will push you to your breaking point, but try to stay on course. Please know in advance that if we finish early, that is nothing to be upset about. Side effects and many complications can hinder your ability to finish the full twelve rounds. Most patients don't make it beyond eight."

"Chemotherapy is a cumulative treatment, and the longer you withstand this treatment, the weaker your body will grow. For many, it won't be safe to continue after a certain point. That is perfectly okay. If we determine you need to stop treatment, we will. Of course, we will hope for more to give you the best fighting chance."

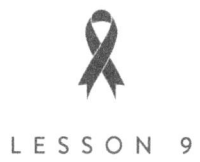

LESSON 9

FIND A WAY TO KEEP GOING

I could write an entire book dedicated to the topic of chemotherapy and the many side effects I endured. You have heard the horror stories, and I don't want to use this book as a place to retell them. Cancer patients are called warriors and fighters for a reason; it takes tremendous courage to bravely show up and continue to push your body to its physical breaking point and what feels like the brink of death.

You never know what may happen, and anything and everything can and often does happen during cancer treatment. I regularly lost control over my body in more ways than you want to know or than I care to share. I've already vulnerably horrified you with ample stories sharing more than enough as it is, but let me reaffirm that chemotherapy not only physically breaks you down but can scare you half to death.

I grew tired of suffering from the severe reactions, and willfully continuing with treatment was hands down one of the hardest things I've ever had to do. It took every ounce of grit to continue going back for more. There were days where my mom and I just sat together in the car outside of the hospital, crying, before she'd help me up and out of the car to finally submit myself to more treatment, despite my wanting nothing more than to give up and quit. If she hadn't been there to whisper how much she loved me and firmly believed in me, and to remind me of all the reasons I wanted to live for Will and the kids, I may not have had the strength to walk into the hospital on more occasions than I care to admit.

It often takes a few rounds of chemotherapy to get used to what to expect and to fully understand how you might respond to receiving treatment. Even after you learn to prepare for commonly experienced reactions, it really never gets any easier.

I could offer plenty of firsthand examples of what I personally experienced, but my point in sharing this with you is to show that you will need to prepare mentally, spiritually, and physically to withstand and persevere. Expect days where even your own power fails you, and you will need someone there to help carry you on.

Your doctor and the infusion center nurses have one goal in mind: treat you and, while doing so, try their best to keep you from suffering any more than necessary. You will likely be prescribed combinations of medications intended to ease common side effects such as nausea, vomiting, and constipation. These are meant to help you be as comfortable as possible, and they do help. I found, though, that the many pharmaceuticals prescribed to treat my chemo reactions could themselves lead to the onset of other side effects and problems, and those could require more drugs to achieve comfort.

It was a vicious cycle. I did learn ways to best prepare for and help tolerate ongoing treatment. These aren't solutions that will make your fight against cancer an easy one, but I do want to share several of the most successful tips and advice that I discovered and personally used that did help me better manage my treatment.

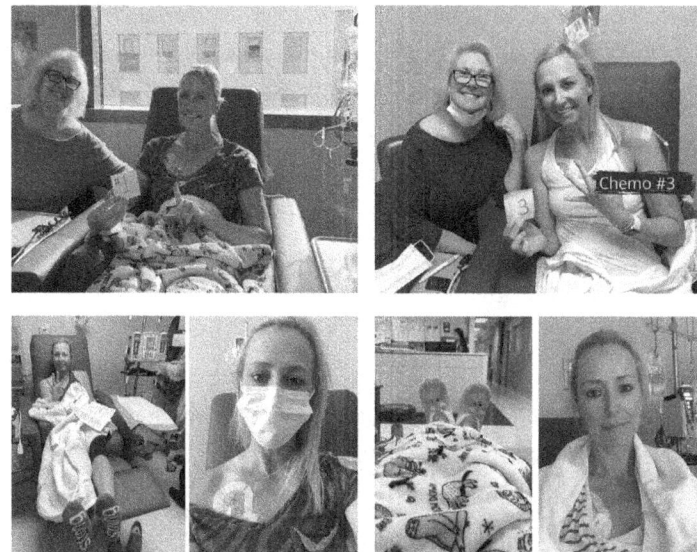

A photo collage from chemotherapy infusions.
Cozy blankets, inspirational socks and my mom for moral support helped.
Shop or donate cancer care bags for patients at authorerinsoto.com.

Nausea and Vomiting

In addition to taking prescribed medications, I was able to ease my nausea and vomiting by changing my eating patterns. On the days that I could stomach food, I ate small meals throughout the day rather than three big ones. I found that apple juice, soothing teas, and ginger ale often helped. Strong smells didn't mix well with nausea, so I avoided pungent foods.

Taste Changes

Some types of chemotherapy can affect your sense of taste. In my case, the temperature of foods or liquids that I was able to tolerate was another factor; anything cold was brutal. I completely lost my appetite for the first few days of each chemo infusion, but it returned within hours after my IV line was taken out. I needed strength and knew I needed to try to eat even while on chemo, but I struggled with this. I would drink warm teas and sip warm soup broth to ensure I was taking in at least a liquid nourishment to help my body recover. Some days liquid was all I could stomach.

The only food that sounded even remotely appetizing during chemo was fresh fruit like papaya or pineapple. I'm not sure why this was the case; maybe because of their natural enzymes and how they soothe the tummy. Whatever the reason, these fruits were my go-to meals during and after chemo treatment infusions.

As you'll find out in the next chapter, I chose to stick to plants like fruits and veggies. Funnily enough, I actually developed a distaste for meat. My body seemed to know and crave exactly what it needed most.

I also always had a slight metallic taste on the tip of my tongue. This is another common reaction to chemotherapy medication. If foods taste metallic, try eating with plastic utensils.

Medications

Talk to your doctor about the best anti-nausea drug for you. Sometimes you may need to try different ones until you find the right version that helps you the most. I required two very strong anti-nauseants which I took, as advised, like clockwork during chemo infusion days. But I found they often led to side effects and discomfort like, among other unpleasantries, severe constipation, making my already-sick self feel even worse. I had to take them but used them only as needed while infusing and during the first few days following, never for as long as was actually prescribed.

What's worse, the many powerful prescription drugs had side effects that then required the help of more prescription drugs. I found myself taking more and more prescription strength meds to treat the side effects of chemotherapy and anti-nauseants. I turned into a pill-popping machine, trying to mask one side effect with a magic pill fix that only led to yet another issue. This made me seek out alternative ways to ease as much of the discomfort as possible without loading up my body with more toxins. I found acupuncture, acupressure, massage, aromatherapy, yoga, and hypnosis helped the most for the strongest side effects. Explore alternative options yourself. You'll be surprised at what works.

Brain Fog

I am going to let you in on another really embarrassing secret. I recently failed a short-term memory test and did so miserably. I wasn't the sharpest tool in the shed before cancer, but now, after chemotherapy, have suffered from the effects of what many refer to as "chemo brain."

My failed memory test was administered by a professional therapist who explained what was to be performed as a "simple exam." All I needed to do in order to pass this test was remember five simple words. Sounds easy enough, right? Wrong! He shared the five words with me and then had me repeat them back to him three times over, to assure I had indeed firmly jogged them into mind. My five words were the following: Alligator. Belt. Glass. Door. Candle.

I asked if I could write the five words down, figuring going into the test that I was probably going to fail. To the average-brained person, this game may seem simple enough. But I already knew how chemo brain had frazzled my short-term memory: I wasn't going to fare well at this easy test. My memory was and still sadly is in very bad shape.

The therapist told me that writing notes would count as cheating; my job was to try my best to just remember the words in my mind. He then successfully distracted my poor feeble brain while carrying on a short conversation, asking first that I recite the last six letters of the alphabet backward and then that I solve several simple mathematical problems.

After only a couple of short minutes had passed, he asked me to recite the five words I was supposed to remember back to him. Only, I couldn't. I tried. I really tried with all my might but could only remember the first two words: alligator and belt.

So sad, right? If we happen to meet in real life someday, please don't bother asking me to remind you about anything important, because chances are I won't remember to remind you. Hard truth! It's not because I'm rude, but because chemo officially has fried my cognitive function. My short-term memory is officially lost, maybe, I am afraid, forever. Thoughts are here one second and gone the very next.

As a busy and active mom of four, my intact memory used to be one of my greatest multi-tasking assets. Losing this superpower makes me sad. Trust me when I say that the struggle is real.

I have found ways to cope. I use my phone to set multiple reminders for when it's time to pick up the kids from school, what items to buy at the grocery store, who to call for an appointment, and many other to-dos I can't seem to recall without organized help and assistance.

Hair Loss

Some, but not all chemo treatments, can lead to hair loss. This is a tough side effect to tolerate because it makes it very obvious to the outside world that you are a cancer patient. People try not to stare, but indeed they do. I hated the looks of pity others often gave me, and having cancer was not something I wanted a constant reminder about every time I looked in the mirror. That can be made more challenging when hair loss is involved.

Thankfully, the colon cancer FOLFOX chemotherapy regimen that I was prescribed sometimes causes only partial hair loss and thinning. It was around chemotherapy round number three when the hunks and chunks of my hair started falling out. I cherished what little hair remained because it was still just enough for me to appear, to those who didn't know me, like I had stringy hair vs. being a cancer patient.

I could still venture out in public and remember, for a brief moment, what it felt like to blend in with everyone else and not be identified as the sickly cancer patient I was. I liked to do this sometimes. I would go somewhere like a supermarket to run an errand and pretend that I was a normal healthy person, like my old self, and try to forget about my having cancer. I would fantasize about the day I could not only play the part of healthy me but might actually feel it, too. I must have gotten good at this because people would seem genuinely shocked when they discovered I was a cancer patient. I guess they expected me to look like I did on the days of, and several days after, I infused chemo.

I was grateful I didn't have total hair loss like many of my cancer friends. I greatly appreciated that I could hide my having cancer when I wanted to, especially on days when I wasn't feeling up to answering the barrage of questions from strangers about what kind of cancer it was, or dealing with the looks and stares that often come from others when they know you are sick. That said, many colon cancer patients on my same chemotherapy regimen do lose all their hair, or so much that they just decide to shave what little remains off anyway.

Shortly after the end of my treatment, during the Coronavirus salon closures, a dear sweet neighbor of mine was doing us a favor by cutting my kids' hair in her garage. Their shaggy hair needed a trim. As she kindly cut and even generously added a little color for the twins' hair requests, she and I discussed my hair loss from having just finished chemotherapy. She then asked me to sit in the salon chair and be her star client, as she had just the idea for a little pick-me-up that could really help.

She used to work at a hair salon and was a color specialist who is still very talented at styling hair. She asked if I wanted to try extensions. She explained to me that she could sew in a strip of hair extensions that she had left over after doing her own hair. Our hair was similar in color, and these were the highest quality to boot. She just so happened to have enough to help fill in my hair loss gaps with what she had on hand. I figured I would give the whole hair extension style a whirl and was thrilled that I did. My hair was instantly transformed back to my pre-cancer long and lustrous appearance. It looked fabulous! I felt fierce.

If your treatment does cause hair loss, here are a few ideas you can consider:

- Use soft-bristle brushes. My hair usually came out after a shower and when I brushed it. Be extra gentle whenever doing this after starting treatment.
- Avoid using hair products with harsh chemicals, and obviously,

avoid hair dyes or permanents. I bought gentle organic shampoo and conditioner and did not color my hair during chemotherapy treatment. It's advisable to wait some time before coloring your hair after treatment; in fact, I waited almost an entire year before I finally felt safe enough to add some highlights to the fragile and slow-growing regrowth I still am working on today. Steer clear of all harsh chemicals during treatment as this will only contribute to hair loss.

- Cutting your hair short may make it look thicker and fuller. Short hair can be super cute and help disguise thinning. I currently am not wearing the hair extensions that my neighbor gifted me. I have since cut my hair short to wear a style that works while I slowly grow my hair loss back.
- Wigs are super stylish now, and you can find high-quality ones that are natural-looking. There are also many programs that specialize in providing wigs to chemo patients at no cost. If you think you'd like a wig, it's suggested that you shop for it before you lose your hair. That way, you can better match it to your hair. Hair loss typically starts to noticeably occur by the second and third rounds of chemotherapy.
- You can wear a head wrap, hat, or scarf. This can look fashionable and obviously also serves a purpose by keeping your head warm, especially during cold weather.
- Your scalp may feel tender and dry. Wash it with mild moisturizing shampoos and conditioners and apply gentle lotions and sunscreen.
- Ice caps were something a few friends recommended to me. One, who is a hairstylist, told me how many of her clients used them successfully to prevent or reduce their hair loss during treatment. You can find different versions of chemo ice caps. I never tried this due to my sensitivity to extreme cold from my potent chemo medication, but I've heard these do really help others who don't suffer the side effects of cold that I did.

- Extensions. If you experience hair thinning rather than complete hair loss, you too can consider using extensions that you either sew or tape in to add volume and length to your hair while it grows back. I used gently sewed in high-quality extensions that didn't cause further damage to the little hair I had left. Be sure to work with a professional and let them know it is important to use high-quality products only that won't tug or pull out your hair if you do decide to try extensions for yourself.

It may sound silly, but after having spent the last eight months hyper-focused on survival, having my hair done that day with extensions was the first time I had done something for my vanity and appearance since having been diagnosed. This little hair moment reminded me that I can and should still do whatever makes me feel great about myself. I had always prided myself in styling my hair and didn't realize how much of my identity I felt I'd lost during treatment after so much of my hair fell out. Feeling like a woman is very important when it comes to confidence, and doing my hair that day gave me a little of my sexy self back.

I followed up my fancy new hairdo with an in-home mani-pedi, my favorite lipstick and some blush, and a date night with the hubby. I was back in action again, tapping into my former girly girl and feeling so great about myself and my looks for the first time since cancer.

Fatigue

Cancer fatigue is real. If you find yourself feeling extremely tired, there are ways to help manage this. Rest or take short naps during the day. Days two to three infusing chemo were often bedridden for me. Focus on conserving your energy for important things and be selective over your reserves. I was highly anemic, and chemotherapy did a number on my blood count. I felt completely drained and was almost always exhausted during cancer treatment. I spent the majority of days two and three while infusing chemo in bed, too weak and sick to move.

After the first round, realizing just how severe my fatigue and general reaction to the infusion could be, our family decided I should stay at my parents' house for a few days after chemo infusions, while Will held down the fort at home.

It certainly didn't help to have a needle and IV line in my chest connected to my chemo pump. This also highly limited movement and made things a little more challenging to work around on top of feeling fatigue. I used chemo infusion days as a time to listen to my body and just allowed myself to rest. Yes, use rest and listen to your body if it tells you to sleep. I napped often and saved up and conserved what limited energy reserve I had. I wanted to remain awake and alert to enjoy visits with Will and the kids. I usually could handle the family visitations for no more than a couple of hours, at most.

That said, exercise is actually considered very good for cancer patients to combat fatigue.

I realize that, after talking about how fatigued I felt, it now will seem counterintuitive to tell you to get out there and move your body. But that is exactly what the doctors will order. There was even a sign hanging in my oncologist's office encouraging cancer patients to exercise.

Exercise is an important part of your cancer treatment plan. A growing amount of research shows that regular exercise can greatly improve physical and mental health during every phase of treatment. Exercise and healing movement also help to boost energy, helping to combat cancer fatigue.

There are many benefits of exercise for cancer patients. Even if you were not active before your cancer diagnosis, an exercise program that meets your unique needs could help you get moving safely and successfully and is something I highly recommend.

You should always speak with your doctor before you start an exercise program during or after cancer treatment. While there are ample exercise forms proven to be safe during different types of cancer treatment, your ability to exercise and the type of exercises you can do will depend on the type of cancer you have and the treatments you are undergoing.

Your current level of fitness obviously needs to be taken into account. This isn't the time to start training for your first marathon, but if you already are an avid runner, some cancer patients continue to run throughout treatment.

I was one of those patients. As a distance runner, I was intrigued by the encouragement to exercise during treatment and asked my oncologist if I would be able to continue running throughout chemotherapy. He told me that as long as I felt physically capable to safely continue doing so, then I had his support to keep on running. He reminded me, however, that my strength and body would be getting broken down as the cumulative effects of treatment took over, and that how I exercised before would likely have to be adjusted in order to safely match my new health condition. My oncologist advised me to keep my heart rate at a safe level and to closely pay attention and listen to the cues my body told me for how far to push myself physically. Play it safe.

That said, the fact that I already ran regularly meant I should be able to continue doing so. Running is almost a form of meditation for me, and I knew I would rely on the physical healing benefits this form of movement always offered me, craving it now more than ever before. I needed to get out into fresh air, clear my mind, and fill my lungs, heart, and body with oxygen while moving to keep my sanity intact.

I found that on day four of a chemo infusion week, the day after I had unplugged, I was ready to get out for a brisk walk. Running at this point was usually too much, too soon. It often felt like I was strapping cinder blocks on my feet in place of my usual running shoes, but that never stopped me from getting out there. Within another day or two, I would go out for a slow and steady jog.

Overall wellbeing

After the first three rounds of chemotherapy got me off to an unusually brutal start, I decided to consider the advice given to me by both my respected and wise fathers. I had been a little reluctant and hesitant at first, as it seemed more like a generationally based suggestion to help treat my grievous cancer symptoms. But it turned out to be sound advice that changed the trajectory of my suffering through treatment.

The solution that helped immensely with my afflicting side effects goes by many names: Mary Jane, pot, grass, cannabis, weed, hemp, hash, marijuana, ganja, and dozens of others. Marijuana is the formal name given to the dried buds and leaves of varieties of the Cannabis sativa plant. I think people need to be educated about the fact that marijuana is not a drug but, rather, an herb.

During my initial consultation with my oncologist, he had asked if we had any questions. My dad thought it was an excellent opportunity to ask Dr. Parker's opinion on the use of medical marijuana to treat the side effects of chemotherapy.

It isn't as though asking the question was that farfetched. In the state of California, marijuana is fully legal, and we all know that many patients have long used medical marijuana to help ease the many discomforts and negative effects commonly experienced with cancer treatment. While this topic may still be a little controversial here today, I would be remiss in writing a book about cancer and not addressing how this wonder herb greatly alleviated my further suffering through the rest of my treatment. It was indeed a turning point and one I recommend and advocate for all cancer patients.

Maybe you have always wondered what smoking weed was like. Now you can find out! And if you happen to have cancer, this is certainly the time in life where nobody should judge you for doing so.

My oncologist acknowledged that while plenty of patients have successfully used cannabis, this wasn't his area of expertise. While he could prescribe THC pills from the pharmacy with my being an active cancer patient, he instead preferred to prescribe me that long list of pharmaceutical drugs to aid with my many side effects.

I started off treatment following his advice, but when those many prescription drugs only led to bigger problems, winding up with me being admitted to the emergency room twice, I decided to consider this more alternative plant-based approach. Both of my dads kept suggesting that I open up my options and consider this a means to help relieve some of my distress. The chemical pills I was being prescribed only seemed to require taking more drugs to treat the new onset of distressing side effects that the last pill had caused, and so I decided to see what all the hype was about.

I was desperate for relief to make my next round of chemotherapy more tolerable, and adamant that I needed to try something different to avoid winding up in the emergency room yet again. I wasn't sure how I could survive the remaining nine rounds of treatment I had left if I couldn't get a hold on easing the many harrowing side effects I was experiencing. Medical marijuana was sounding more and more appealing. I did my own research and found a string of reports on the benefits of its use.

My dad had suggested it was high time (pun intended) for my first field trip to a local dispensary to meet with a local "potista" and inquire about what might be of help for someone in my situation. A potista is a budtender, similar to a bartender, or to a barista at a coffee shop. A potista is someone who has all the 411 you will ever need to know about 420. They are experts on the various forms and can suggest or offer advice if this is something new to you.

I explained to the potista that as a mom of four and active cancer patient, I needed something on the strong side to help during the most sick and uncomfortable days when I was infusing chemo. And for the days after infusions, I needed another less strong version that could continue to ease discomfort, pain, and anxiety but still allow me to fully function coherently as a mom. There were options.

As a nonsmoker, I prefer to use oil drops and edibles. Smoked marijuana can deliver harmful substances to users, including many of the same substances found in tobacco smoke. I wanted only the medicinal plant-based benefits, but without the harmful inhalation of smoke.

Talk to your doctor about what you should expect when taking one of these herbal drugs and what negative side effects may be caused by other medication you are taking. It's a good idea to have someone with you when you first start testing medical marijuana. Have them be there after any dosage changes as well.

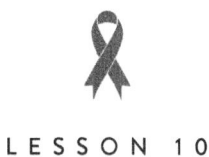

LESSON 10

THINK ABOUT WHAT YOU PUT IN YOUR BODY

When I asked my medical team of experts for direction regarding cancer and diet following my diagnosis, I was disappointed with their responses. I was basically told to continue eating the very same foods I had formerly enjoyed as soon as I recovered from my surgery. The same foods? Like beer and chips? Like red meat and sugary sweets? Really?

That certainly didn't settle right with me. I instinctively knew that there had to be more of a link between the foods I was eating and my developing advanced colorectal cancer, cancer that was quite literally located inside of my digestive tract. Talk about location, location, location!

I refused to accept their "eat whatever you like" answer and decided to investigate more into the connection between nutrition and illness. Thankfully, I didn't have to look far to find answers. There are ample resources out there pertaining to cancer and diet, and experts from those resources all provide similar suggestions and guidance. My favorites are *Crazy Sexy Kitchen* by Kris Carr and Chef Chad Sarno and *Cancer-Free With Food* and *The Earth Diet,* both by Liana Werner-Gray.

Up until my diagnosis our family had been following a paleo diet, consuming high amounts of clean meat under the false assumption that this was the best way for us to stay fit and healthy. After all, it's what our ancestors ate, right? I also was told a paleo diet was the best one to follow for my daughter's autoimmune disease. I even read countless books about chronic inflammation, leaky gut and autoimmune disorders, all suggesting paleo was the best solution.

I believed that I was making an informed diet decision in the best interest of my family. It turns out I was likely contributing to the various health problems we all were suffering from, my cancer included. That is a very frightening thought to digest now.

The last thing I wanted to do was continue eating the same foods that I had been eating prior to my cancer diagnosis and expect a different result. That is the very definition of insanity.

Among the majority of trusted experts within the cancer community, there seems to be a shared consensus for best practices around healing cancer through nutrition. In fact, in the couple of years since I was diagnosed and began researching cancer and diet, the same answers I discovered have since become widely accepted across the industry. I am very happy to report that my healthcare provider has since provided me with research on using a plant-based diet to combat disease and improve health.

Practically all the latest scientific research and cancer diet books that I read suggest four primary dietary changes:

- Reduce or eliminate meat, dairy, sugar, and refined foods
- Significantly increase fruit and vegetable intake
- Eat organic
- Drink plenty of clean filtered water

The bulk of the latest research supports eating less meat with a lot more evidence on how moving towards a plant-based diet may help.

Cancer is the second-leading cause of death in the U.S., but estimates suggest that as many as a third of cases could be prevented with diet and nutrition alone.[1] Let me repeat that last line again for the people in the back: estimates suggest that as many as a third of cases could be prevented with diet and nutrition alone. That is empowering information according to a recent article by The Mayo Foundation for

Medical Education and Research which is one of the most respected academic medical center organizations in America.

Why Not Meat?

Fun Fact: Vegetarians have significantly lower cancer rates.[2] In the largest study recently performed on an anti-cancer diet, the European Prospective Investigation into Cancer and Nutrition-Oxford (EPIC-Oxford) concluded that the overall incidence of all cancers combined is lower among vegetarians. I should add that vegans fared even better.[3]

A study done by Drs. Dean Ornish and Nobel Prize winner Elizabeth Blackburn concluded that a vegan diet caused more than 500 genes to change in only three short months, turning on genes that prevent disease and turning off genes that cause breast cancer, heart disease, prostate cancer, and many other illnesses.[4]

Research suggests a link between meat and cancer. In one review, each additional 3.5 ounces of red meat a day raised the relative risk of colorectal polyps by 2%. Just half as much daily processed meat — such as deli meats or hot dogs — raised the risk by 29%.

Dr. Kelly Turner's *Radical Remission* book reports that eating just two servings of meat each day quadrupled a woman's risk of breast cancer recurrence. Quadrupled the risk of recurrence! That just made me squirm in my seat as I typed it. It is precisely why, now, I continue to avoid consuming very much meat.

Why do vegans and vegetarians have such lower cancer risks?[5] The answer is rather fascinating. A study of the Pritikin experiments putting people on a plant-based diet along with exercise show that in as little as 12 days they can turn their bloodstream into a cancer cell fighting machine.[5] A series of experiments, performed to see whose diet kicked the most cancer butt, also displayed very significant results. People were placed on various diets and then had their blood dripped on human cancers cells growing inside of a petri dish. Here is what they found.

Women who were placed on a plant-based diet for only two short weeks were able to suppress the growth of three different types of breast cancer. What is more, their bodies gained the power to substantially slow down - and even stop - cancer cell growth.[6] This all occurred after only TWO WEEKS of going vegan. Similar results were achieved with men in the same study for prostate cancer. Imagine what you can accomplish after several months following a vegan diet, or better yet, after an entire year.

How can a simple dietary change make someone's blood averse to cancer on a cellular level and do so in just a matter of days? The improvement in cancer defense that was measured after two weeks of eating plant-based is believed to be due to changes in the level of a cancer-promoting growth hormone found in your body called Insulin-like growth factor (IGF-1).[7]

IGF-1 is a natural human growth hormone that is instrumental in normal growth during your childhood, but in adulthood it can promote abnormal growth—the spread, metastasis, and invasion of cancer cells.

Animal protein, that is, meat and dairy products, increases the levels of IGF-1 in your body. The good news is that if you are only just discovering the science of how this all works when reading this here today, it is not too late. As the studies have proven, just two weeks of switching to a plant-based diet can lead to your IGF-1 levels dropping low enough to help slow down, and even stop, the growth of cancer.

That is some impressive power, found simply by eating more plants. This research and plentiful success stories the world over, from many who claim the vegan diet drastically helped them in their fight against cancer, resulted in my diving all-in, going 100% vegan for eight months immediately following my diagnosis. I wanted to regain some sense of control over my disease and figured that cutting out meat and dairy was a tactical defense strategy I could easily follow in my personal fight to beat cancer.

After announcing our pro-plant love, we requested that only vegetarian and vegan dinners be delivered to our family through the meal train friends had set up to assist during my treatment. The questions around dietary concerns immediately started rolling in.

My own beloved mother, a member of a multigenerational family of Arizona cattle ranchers, seemed particularly worried that this veggie transition might be detrimental to our health.

Newsflash! There are no magical nutrients found in meat that you cannot get from other plant-based sources.

I began posting videos and photos of the kids helping me prepare our new plant-based meals. I found myself answering questions from many curious friends about how the foods we were now eating were meeting the dietary needs of all members in our household if they all excluded meat. The question most often asked was whether we would get our sufficient intake of protein from eating plants alone.

Many falsely assumed this change could make my body grow weaker during cancer treatment, when I needed strength, causing further harm from a lack of sufficient nutrients. They were also concerned that it could stunt my children's growth.

Here is how I best explained this to those new to the vegan and vegetarian movement: Some of the most respected professional athletes, as well as many Olympians, measure their performance through clinical and scientific research. Studies found that those who have adopted plant-based diets went into optimal physical achievement as a direct result of their vegan diet.

The Game Changers, a popular documentary, came out around the same time we were starting this diet transition in our household. I suggested to many that they watch the show, as it explained this concept in an entertaining way and made the information easy to grasp. If you haven't heard about or seen this yet for yourself, I highly recommend watching it.

Back to the protein concern. Fun Fact: Plant-based diet eaters get 70% more protein than they need.[8] There's the answer you can give to those posing concerned inquiries about your getting sufficient protein from plants.

All protein originates in plants. The protein that you get from eating a steak or a burger is actually coming from the plants that the animal ate. So, no, you don't need a hunk of meat on your plate as your staple for protein. What you really need is a mouthful of protein-rich plants. In fact, whether they realize it or not, most meat-eaters get more than half of their protein from plants.

Plants naturally produce phytochemicals that protect your cells from damage. Phytochemicals have a long list of beneficial effects, including preventing cancer. They also help your body recuperate from intense physical exercise or damage caused by cancer treatment.

Vegan athletes often note that they recover more quickly than when they consumed meat. I can vouch for that. I was often asked how on earth I was up and literally running the day after my 48-hour chemotherapy infusions. I know that my vegan diet allowed me to bounce back more quickly from cancer treatment because I was fueling my body to protect from the damage caused to it.

If going fully vegan or vegetarian still seems too daunting for you, I understand. I personally did so for myself because the statistics relating to cancer were promising and encouraging enough for me to believe that a vegan diet would best support my effort to survive.

I went vegan for eight months and, coincidentally, went into remission during my vegan period. I continue to primarily eat vegan and vegetarian to this day but admit that I now permit myself the occasional cheat day. I will cheat for holidays, vacations, and dinner parties. Keep in mind that moderation is key, and cheating is not the norm.

I don't actually crave the same foods today that I used to before going vegan. And I often feel sick if I eat too much animal product, which helps me stick with my healthier new dietary preference.

That said, I allowed my family to continue eating meat, but substantially less, rather than fully eliminating it. They went on a slow transition as I went all-in cancer-crushing vegan. They stuck to poultry or fish a couple of times a week. My best advice is just do whatever you can tolerate. It all adds up and will matter. Eating a plant-based diet doesn't have to be all or nothing. Even small changes can still make a major impact.

The Dairy Debate

Dairy has been an area of controversy for a long time. Many studies have examined the relationship between dairy consumption and cancer. Some studies indicate that dairy may protect against cancer, while others suggest that dairy may increase cancer risk. Virtually all studies on the connection between milk and cancer are observational in nature, that is, they cannot prove that dairy products cause disease, only that consuming dairy is associated with it.

Some studies suggest an arguable point as to why reducing dairy from your diet is advised: All dairy products are made from the breast milk of another animal. Cows' milk is an example. A mama cow's milk is jam-filled with hormones and proteins designed by nature to help her baby calf grow. Cow's milk was never intended for human consumption. Let's just leave that there for you to consider a moment more.

In many cases, what cows feed on often affects the nutritional quality and health properties of their milk. A recent study out of California's Loma Linda University showed a strong correlation between cow's milk and higher breast cancer rates, a link previously considered unfounded by most experts. While the study suggests an association with breast cancer risk, it does not say that milk directly causes the disease.

The way I came to view this hot topic is that vegetarians who consume dairy still benefit overall from reduced cancer rates in comparison to those who consume meat.

Milk and dairy are also reliable sources of calcium and protein and are considered by many to be part of a healthy balanced diet. I would be remiss in not highlighting that there has also been convincing evidence linking milk to a decrease in colorectal cancer risk.

The bottom line is that we are vulnerable to anything we eat. The amount of fat (particularly saturated fat), salt, and sugar in dairy products can vary. I opt for healthier low-fat, low-sugar dairy products, and often use dairy alternatives that help maintain a healthy weight, reducing my risk for cancer.

The research to date on dairy consumption and cancer has been inconsistent. I believe that moderation is always the key. I avoid excessive consumption of dairy products. My general approach has been to stick to reducing the consumption of dairy, mixing it up by using other kinds of plant-based dairy alternatives. For example, in place of milk, I often use almond milk, cashew milk, hemp milk, oat milk, or rice milk. I also prefer plant-based butter and cream in place of the heavy high-fat dairy versions. Dairy alternatives are also excellent sources of calcium.

Similar to the argument that you don't need milk for calcium, despite the commercials many of us grew up watching telling us all that "milk does our body good," is that, like meat, dairy products do not provide you with any nutrients that you cannot get elsewhere. Like from eating a plateful of iron- and calcium-rich plants, such as leafy greens, beans, and nuts.

Sweet as Sugar

During my paleo diet I had already cut most refined carbohydrates and sugar from my diet, so this change wasn't a drastic one to commit to on my part.

There are many studies about sugar and cancer that are readily available through a quick internet search. There's also a lot of confusing and misleading information. That's unfortunate because there is important science to understand.

The connection made between sugar and cancer was first discovered back in 1920 when Nobel Peace Prize Dr. Otto Warburg basically concluded, in layman's terms, that cancer cells behave much differently from healthy cells and require high amounts of sugar in order to function.

Although research has shown that cancer cells consume more sugar than normal cells, no studies have shown that eating sugar will make your cancer worse or that, if you avoid eating sugar, your cancer will disappear.

What is the link between sugar and cancer? Refined sugar can affect your body in different ways, including increasing the risks of obesity, heart disease, and diabetes; and it impacts your energy, mood, and dental health.

There is no question that obesity is associated with an increased risk of cancer and that the abundance of carbohydrates in our diet is one of the major foundations on which the worldwide obesity epidemic is built.

Body fat promotes inflammation, which can damage DNA and lead to cancer. Eating lots of refined carbohydrates, including foods with added sugar, can lead to excess weight gain, which is associated with an increased risk of developing several types of cancer.

Does the body need sugar to survive? Yes, your body needs it for energy, but you need to give it the right kind and consider the source. The body breaks down all carbohydrates into glucose. Naturally occurring sugars come with a variety of nutrients that the body needs to stay healthy. For example, along with fructose, fruits contain fiber and various vitamins and minerals.

However, according to the American Heart Association (AHA), the body doesn't need added sugar, such as the sugar in soda, for survival. Processed and refined sugar is not good for your health.

Manage your weight by eating a balanced diet, avoiding too many refined carbohydrates that lack fiber and foods with added sugars. That is my best diet advice for diet and cancer.

Drink More Water

Some theorize that drinking water with a higher pH can increase your metabolism and will help your body improve its ability to absorb vital nutrients. It's believed it will help starve any cancer cells found in your body, because cancer cells thrive in an acidic environment.

Water is essential for proper hydration of your cells, tissues, and organs, as well as being your primary means of eliminating toxins. A great rule of thumb is to aim to drink half your body weight in ounces of water per day. If you are in active cancer treatment, your medical care team will elaborate further about the many reasons you need to increase your water consumption to help you recover from cancer treatment. Chemotherapy is highly dehydrating. You'll be advised to, following a cycle of chemotherapy, flush out the chemicals to avoid dehydration and decrease common cancer treatment side effects.

We all well know that water is just plain ol' good for you. In fact, up to 60% of the human adult body is actually water. Your brain and heart are composed of 73% water, the lungs are about 83% water, your skin is 64% water, muscles and kidneys are 79%, and even your bones are about 31% water!

I really shouldn't need to elaborate on why you need to prioritize staying fully hydrated to maintain optimum health. Feel free to look this up if you want to learn more, but drinking water is super simple to do more of. Drink up, Buttercup - and cheers!

I suggest the following guidelines for cancer and diet: maintain a healthy weight; be physically active; properly hydrate with water; eat a diet rich in vegetables, fruit, whole grains, and beans; avoid refined carbohydrates, including foods with added sugar; limit red meat and stay away from processed meat or, ideally, try to eliminate meat altogether; and avoid alcohol.

I followed my above advice and filled up on plant-based foods for the year I actively had cancer. Now that I am in remission, I try to keep to the occasional poultry or fish meal, limiting this to once and maybe twice a week, tops. I strictly apply the 80/20 rule in our home. While I allow my family to eat a little meat here and there, I often still prepare a vegan or vegetarian alternative dinner for myself and any others who prefer the option. I try to always have some plant-based leftovers or another dish readily available.

My son Cristian chose to go vegan along with me, and he's really committed to his diet. He watched everything that I went through during cancer and wants to put himself in the best position to avoid developing this disease himself in the future.

Well-meaning family members share their strong opinions about Cristian's strict aversion to meat and dairy, saying he's acting out of fear. On the contrary, I view his decision as an empowering one, one that he is making for his personal health and something for which he ought to be praised, not criticized. To decide this at his young age of twelve years is commendable, something many grown adults don't have the willpower to commit to for themselves.

Since all of my children are at an increased risk for developing colorectal cancer, they will require screening starting in their twenties. Our all eating mostly vegetarian and vegan was that much more important to instill in them considering their hereditary risk factor. It is a powerful preventative move we could all make together and one I wanted them to learn to transition to.

Going completely vegan may seem intimidating, extreme, and difficult if you are anything like we were. It's especially true if you happen to have miniature picky eaters at your dinner table. The vegan diet was something I knew I personally could easily transition over to. My kids, well, that was going to be tricky.

I had been a vegan and vegetarian back in the day, during high school and early college years, following in the footsteps of my older brother, Scott, who has been vegan since he was a teen and has remained so throughout his adult life. In other words, I was somewhat well-versed through personal experience and family exposure. My kids and husband, however, were not. Not by a long shot! They moaned and groaned and didn't at all fully embrace the initial announcement of our transition, but they were also motivated and wanted to support my cancer journey. We had a family talk, and all committed to this change together.

One of the ways I helped to make this transformation easier for my family was to involve everyone in the weekly meal prep and planning. We tested out a lot of recipes for several months before identifying those that qualified as new family favorites, earning a coveted spot in our weekly rotation of repeat dinners.

The kitchen in our home is where the hustle and bustle of the day come to a pause. It's the place where we can gather together, recount stories from our day and work on homework, all while chopping, simmering, and filling our home with the scents of a delicious family meal.

I HOPE THIS HELPS

Making this kind of a drastic change, especially with kids involved, is all about finding balance. To shift to a more plant-based diet that you'll all actually enjoy and want to stick with, I suggest making this a gradual change. Some tips to help:

Start Slow. Cut out one meat, dairy, sugar, or refined food every day. Explore healthier options to replace those. Try vanilla-flavored oat milk for your coffee creamer. Substitute honey, agave, or maple syrup for refined white sugar, or try using coconut sugar instead.

Experiment with meatless meals. Set a goal of trying one to two brand new meat-free recipes a week. Keep a list of the winners and continue testing new recipes until you acquire a list of meals that made the family cut. Shoot for at least a couple of weeks' worth of dinners, then rotate through them routinely, easing off the adventurous testing of new food for a while to perfect the winners you have all come to love.

Create a food rating sheet. Make the taste test phase a fun experiment for the whole family to get in on. Identify the winners by allowing everyone to eat and then, at the table, rate the new veggie dinners together.

Eat at least one serving of fruit or vegetable with every meal. Gradually increase fruits and vegetables until half of your plate is filled with them.

Prioritize buying organic. If you continue to consume meat and dairy, buy only the cleanest, healthiest versions. And when it comes to produce, you should research the dirty dozen and learn which fruits and vegetables carry the most pesticides: apples, celery, tomatoes, etc. Use a homemade or purchased cleansing wash for your produce to remove wax and pesticides.

Bonus Savings: In time, as you start to cut down (or out) on the costly meat, eating more fruits, vegetables, and plant proteins, even with organic costing a bit more, you should notice that your monthly grocery expense is less than before.

Try investing in a juicer. After a few weeks of transitioning to more fruits and veggies, you should start experimenting with more smoothies and then consider graduating up to juicing your favorite vegetables and fruit juices.

Try the 7-day plant-based challenge. During this time, you must eliminate all dairy, meat, non-fruit sugar, eggs, gluten, soy, alcohol, and caffeine. This isn't too long of a time period to seem daunting; it is actually very doable. Notice how you feel, by the end of the seven days, in energy level and vitality. Then, if you want, you may slowly start to reintroduce foods you cut out, one by one, being careful to space them every three to five days. You might learn which foods cause you to feel worse after eating and, can, if you wish, cut those out.

Cheat Days Will Help You Stick With It. I've admitted that I am a cheater. My kids and family will warn you never to play cards with me. I do cheat at some things I do, and this certainly applies to my diet. I plan to cheat on vacations and holidays, knowing I will intentionally go off my usual clean dietary routine, but somehow it helps me stick with the bigger picture of a healthier diet the rest of the time.

For more tips and meal plans, visit my website, **www.authorerinsoto.com**

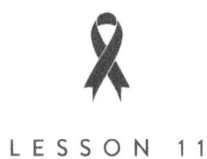

LESSON 11

THINK ABOUT WHAT YOU PUT ON YOUR BODY

Prior to my diagnosis, I prided myself on being what I considered a responsible and safe shopper. I thought I had been making clean decisions for my family, but I discovered that many of the items we often used failed the toxicity test.

I'm talking about common products that you also may have easily overlooked, from your kitchen counter cleaning spray, laundry and dishwasher detergents to your hair conditioner, body lotion, toothpaste, and deodorant—plus many more.

I was unaware of how much I was doing wrong and wish someone had helped me learn how to identify ways to better champion protection on behalf of my family. After I examined the pervasive use of toxic chemicals found in many of these common products, I was appalled.

I was guilty of buying into deceiving marketing ploys used by popular brands, believing they were safe simply because their packaging told me so.

Spoiler alert! Many are not.

In order to meet the rising consumer demand for safer ingredients, some companies have attempted to mislead you with clever use of marketing and packaging. The products, at first blush, appear to be free of harmful ingredients; in fact, they are still dangerously dirty.

I was astounded to discover just how badly the cosmetics industry is under-regulated –it seems even more so than our food and drug sectors. They say oblivion is bliss. Well, I blissfully applied copious amounts of those not-so-pure lotions, potions, and cosmetics to my skin for years.

I'm a self-professed girly girl. One of my very first jobs back in high school was working for several well-known global cosmetic lines at a department store cosmetic section. I continued this, using and selling beauty products at the various manufacturer's counters, throughout college.

I thought I was lucky to work as a beauty insider. I loved the creams, makeup, and goodies I was gifted by the cosmetic beauty lines. Self-testing the products helped me recommend them to shoppers. Looking back, I started exposing my body to many carcinogens when I was just a teenager.

The repeated daily exposure I have had with many products over all these years is a disturbing thought. This includes items I more recently purchased for my family members, ones that I have since discovered included hormone-disrupting chemicals and toxic substances.

Cancer was the tipping point for me to finally open my eyes to the dangers. I embraced making a much-needed change in an effort to better protect myself, and more importantly, those I love.

I had never considered that my favorite lip balm or my children's baby lotion and bubble bath (containing formaldehyde) was dangerous, but that was indeed the case. I shudder, reflecting on the damage I might have caused to my children. It is infuriating.

If you are equally upset after reading this for yourself, you ought to be. We have all been paying others to poison our bodies over an entire lifetime of dangerous product use and consumption. We have blindly been placing our trust in companies who have been putting our health in harm's way for the sake of profit.

Fret not, as help has arrived. This won't require your having to memorize lengthy names of the many chemical ingredients that you now need to avoid, nor must you read books and conduct all of the research I completed in order to safely proceed. I encourage you to do so if learning interests you; but, for the sake of what you need to do now, this is far easier than it appears.

I'm going to let you in on one of my not-so-dirty (pun intended) little secrets. One that you can use immediately to start protecting yourself and your family today. There is a simple tool that you can use to quickly identify truly clean and safe products moving forward. It is an app that my clean living and environmentally conscious older brother introduced me to called Think Dirty.

The app educates and empowers consumers by allowing us to make informed decisions on products that are the safest option to purchase. It helps consumers identify potential risks associated with the many products that you use every day. It does so in a matter of seconds with the click of a button on your smartphone.

I should add that I am in no way affiliated with Think Dirty. I just am a huge fan and tell everyone that I know all about this resource. It is one of my most favorite apps on my phone.

This app allows consumers to learn about potentially toxic ingredients found in products by letting you perform a quick safety test. When you scan the barcode, the app generates a score rating on the dirty meter. Products range from being red and dirty, to yellow and half n' half, to the best level of green and clean.

I use the app while shopping in stores, scanning the barcodes for every new product I am considering purchasing to first learn its safety rating. You can also perform a search for items without scanning their barcode if you don't have the product in hand to scan directly.

You can easily assess the overall risk of thousands of products based on the potential health impact of every listed ingredient. With the app, you don't have to become a label reading expert. It will quickly do the work for you.

After my cancer diagnosis, I'll admit I became a little obsessed with using the app because of how fun and simple it was to use. Sometimes the results were shocking. We were in the midst of moving when I first went through my entire home, scanning practically every bottle I could get my hands on, tossing out all toxic items I felt landed too low on the safety scale for my family to continue using.

Not only does this break down every single ingredient for you, both offensive and clean, it also educates you as to why the product ranks where it does on their dirty scale. So many items throughout my house that were deceivingly labeled as clean and free of chemicals turned out to be full of toxic and dangerous ingredients. The app is fascinating to learn from and a little addictive to use. Enjoy scanning as your next homework assignment.

I HOPE THIS HELPS

Your turn! Time to clean house. Download the Think Dirty App and start checking the ranking for items throughout your home to quickly determine how safe your products are. Throw away items you can part with that fall below your comfort level on the dirty scale. While shopping for better alternatives to replace what you tossed, scan barcodes. Start to make the transition to a healthier household.

While the app allows you to shop on it for their suggested clean products, many of these items can be found on major online retailers and at your local department store. So, use the app to suggest products and brands that have a safe reputation and ranking, then add them to your shopping list.

PART IV

How to Heal the Soul

LESSON 12

Know When To Let Go

During that wild month of November, while everything seemed to be happening all at once, I had the bright idea of visiting a life coach and spiritual advisor to seek consolation that all was going to be okay.

There was a lot to process at the time: selling our house and packing it up, Will's announcement to resign from his job, the new nonprofit I'd been working on starting up, plans to prepare for our big move to Costa Rica that summer, the lawsuit, and financial hits we had taken.

I felt we could benefit from some guidance, counseling, therapy, or direction from an outsider with an objective perspective.

I know that, for some, reading what I'm about to delve into will seem a little out of left field and possibly will even be a new concept you haven't been introduced to yet. I can relate because I was incredibly skeptical and struggled over embracing self-development and spirituality practices in my own life for many years.

I would hate to lose you in this chapter because this may not resonate with you. I have decided to share individual stories in this book that will touch upon common themes many self-growth gurus, popular influencers, and thought provokers preach.

I do not consider myself anywhere near being an expert in teaching these concepts; I am a student myself. But I am comfortable enough sharing stories about things I've directly tested out in my life that you might think are a bit crazy. What I learned has value to me. It may carry lessons everyone should consider for their journey to health and happiness.

I simply ask in advance that you please try to keep an open mind, even if this is something you do not believe in. If you've never heard of the concept before and are cautious about what I'm suggesting you try in this chapter, I encourage you to continue reading and take it in, even if you don't follow through on the actionable step I'm proposing.

Fair warning: the way I went about seeking help may come across as unusual to you. It seemed a bit so to me at first. But stay with me. I assure you that even if the source of advice I used isn't what you would choose to personally seek help for yourself, at the very least you will enjoy the entertainment factor. The lessons I learned might apply to you and your healing, regardless of where I gathered the insight from.

Spiritual health is part of healing the mind, body, and soul. We've covered the first two sides of that triangle. Please stick with me while we tackle the last.

After years of being devoted to personal development as a way to work through the mid-life stressors that Will and I had been experiencing, I finally accomplished processing the years of setbacks and let go of the bitterness and suffering I had become accustomed to living with and seemed stuck in a cycle of repeating.

Years ago, a friend of my husband had told him she regularly visits a spiritual life coach in Carlsbad, California. She swore up and down that he needed to see this coach, that she was the "real deal" and had been a tremendous help to her after her mom had passed away. She insisted he go in for an appointment.

Will went. He came home and recounted many details about our private life that this lady somehow had picked up on and offered guidance for, topics she had no way of possibly knowing about. My husband didn't offer the information, yet she never-the-less narrowed in on the issues we most needed to work on. Will went in as a skeptic and came out as a firm believer that she was indeed a life coach with a legitimate spiritual gift.

Wanting to disprove this, thinking that she must have researched our family on social media or found out what she knew about my husband through some explicable source, I booked an appointment to see for myself. My first meeting with Janet was right after we had lost our home, back in 2008, moving in with my mother-in-law after our twins were born.

I intended to prove my husband wrong, showing that Janet somehow had pulled off a magnificent ploy. But within five minutes of meeting with her myself, I had to insert my foot into my mouth and own up to my limited thinking and mindset.

The day before my appointment, I had just accepted a job offer from The Walt Disney Company. Nobody other than Will was aware of this. When they recently met, Will had not mentioned to Janet my interview and consideration of a new job opportunity. Not even my sister had heard the news about my accepting my new position.

When I sat down, the very first thing she said was how she didn't quite know how to make sense of what she was seeing, but for some reason, she was being shown a vision of Mickey Mouse. I nearly fell out of my chair in disbelief. She thought it was strange to see the cartoon character and asked if possibly we had recently visited Disneyland. I confirmed this was actually because I had just accepted an offer to start working for the company.

During our first meeting, through her incredible predictions and insight, Janet shared many surprisingly accurate revelations that would come to fruition. I continue to visit her every year to check in for further guidance. I always enjoy the advice she shares. It comes from someone who genuinely cares, who, as a life coach, has my best interests at heart. I consider her accuracy in predicting future events an added perk.

During one of my appointments, Janet told me that she doesn't often tell people this, but she had seen my husband and me living very happily with our family. She saw us in a beautiful home with a rainbow over it, which meant we were going to have a long and peaceful life together.

She even teared up when she shared that, explaining she doesn't get to say promising news to everyone with whom she meets. Doing so brought her joy. On my part, it was reassuring.

Will and I decided to go in for an appointment together just before Thanksgiving in 2019, hoping Janet could offer us some positive news about the never-ending lawsuit ordeal, as well as advice about our big plans for the international move. What she predicted instead absolutely boggled my mind.

We wanted her to tell us the lawsuit was coming to an end, that she saw Will landing a job and our family relocating to Costa Rica. Instead, she explained to Will that his leaving real estate for a job in lending wasn't the right path for him.

She reminded him of how great he was at his job when he didn't have to worry or feel pressure about where his business would be generated from. When his primary role was to focus on servicing his clients, he excelled and enjoyed his work.

She advised against a career transition, suggesting, instead, that a simple change in the company environment he worked in was a better solution. She told him not to give up hope and that something indeed would work out for the better in the coming months.

His homework was to remain focused on the parts of his job that he liked most, to bring more of that into fruition with his next job, and to stop focusing on all that wasn't working well. Janet warned that not doing so would attract more of what he did not want. The right job would be coming soon. And indeed, as you know, it was just around the corner.

As we shared with her what else was going on with our lawsuit and financial struggles, mostly intent on talking about Will during the meeting, Janet noticeably shifted her attention to me.

• • •

When we typically visit Janet, she's calm and smiling. Our meetings have always started with small talk and happy conversation. This was different from business as usual. As we began to share updates about our legal troubles, she interrupted us both, saying we could get to that later. First, she felt a need to talk with me about concerns over my health.

She said that when I had entered her office on this day, she became genuinely worried. She explained that my aura was not its usual color; rather, in fact, it was completely black, which is not a good sign.

What was worse, there seemed to be some form of black mass flowing out from my lower abdominal area. She described it as being toxic, very negative, and dangerous. She said this mass was trickling outward, surrounding every part of my body, sucking away my energy and poisoning my health.

I laughed, explaining that we thought there were some pesky parasites in my digestive tract, nothing major to worry about. Janet wasn't convinced. She said the pain I had experienced from the legal and financial hardships had made me physically ill. I explained to her how deeply I had been hurt and upset over everything happening to our family, to the extent that I had recently suffered from a nervous breakdown, with several severe panic attacks and extreme anxiety.

I said I figured the best way to work through all of that was to find forgiveness for those doing this to us. I believed I could free myself from the physiological angst and mental impact this experience had on me if only I could find it in my heart to forgive the people intent on inflicting harm on my family for financial gain.

I told her how I believe that nobody is born evil or greedy. People like this must have lost their way through their own life experiences. I wanted to understand better how they came to view the world, how they had grown willing to hurt our family. I thought that then I could forgive.

I admitted I was practically obsessed with this, and noted I often sought guidance to do so in the form of prayer. I thought that if I could view them as the sum of their negative life experiences, I could make enough sense of their actions to find peace within myself. Janet explained to me how doing this had been a horrible mistake and was a dangerous move on my part.

"You have been going about this in the wrong way. You will never understand people like this. Their energy, unlike yours, is negative." she said. "You don't need to sink to their level or try to understand in order to forgive them."

She explained that I would never understand what they have done because I exist in a different reality from them. How I view the world in comparison to how they see it is like night and day. I hold a higher perspective and cannot commit acts they do, without care or consciousness.

My desperate effort to try to forgive them through prayer had somehow created a toxic psychic bond. Now their negative energy was harming me more than the emotional and financial pain caused to us. She insisted I was becoming physically sick due to this dangerous psychic connection.

She never said I had cancer, but practically implied it by referring to this as "soul cancer." My tuning in to all this negativity was manifesting physically inside of my body. I apparently was dangerously ill. I would come to discover, one week later, that the invisible black mass Janet saw protruding from my lower abdomen was in the exact location of my tumor, and that I had colorectal cancer.

Janet asked me to explain more about my stomach problems.

I was so surprised by her accuracy. I tried to assure her my digestive troubles were nothing to be worried about. She was convinced otherwise, so much so that she grabbed my hands, looked me straight in the eyes, and insisted I pay close attention to what she wanted me to do immediately after our meeting.

Years ago, she had been studying in India on a spiritual retreat. One of her fellow attendees was a highly regarded Native American shaman. He taught her about spiritual cleansing bath rituals that could help cleanse the aura and energy from negative connections or psychic attacks, much like the one she felt I was experiencing. This was only to be used for emergencies, which she considered the invisible black mass to be.

At the time of our meeting I still wasn't fully convinced, but I agreed to follow her directions. I promised to take a spiritual cleansing bath and use her suggested safe version of a prayer of forgiveness.

She wrote down the ingredients for the bath and the directions for my prayer, the proper way to forgive in place of how I had wrongly been going about doing it. She suggested I do this several times over the next couple of weeks and then continue monthly as needed.

She explained that I needed to visualize the invisible psychic cords coming out of my abdomen and connecting me to this negative energy, and to see myself cutting these chords, thus breaking the connection. After I had completed this, I was supposed to visualize myself being completely cleansed from head to toe, surrounded by a bright white light clearing my aura.

Will and I got into our car and looked at one another, giggling about this energy we couldn't see that was supposedly encompassing and poisoning my body. Not so funny, looking back. As usual, she was spot on and, once again, I'm left in complete awe of her spiritual gift and am a firm believer that she really knows her stuff. She knew I had cancer before I was ever diagnosed.

When we got home later that night I ran my bath, but admit I treated this more like a mommy spa night because I wasn't taking it to heart. I still thought we were talking about parasites here, not cancer.

During my spa soak, Will came into the bathroom with my youngest, Liam, who wanted to join me for my fancy bubble bath time. I was embarrassed that Will and he had interrupted me acting like a hippie, woo-woo, bohemian rhapsody nutcase; so, I didn't really follow through as instructed on my first round.

I had lit candles around the counter for aromatherapy and was relaxing to a playlist of spa and meditation sounds. But I ended up turning the first spiritual bath into a playdate with Liam, adding bubbles to the water and failing to properly follow directions.

After being diagnosed with cancer a week later, you'd better believe I took another Native American shaman cleansing bath. This time though, I fully committed my intention to the effort. The week following my diagnosis Janet's words continued to haunt my mind. I was desperate and willing to try anything that could help heal me, no matter how bizarre or silly it sounded.

If someone told me that climbing a tree in the remote rainforest whilst hanging upside down from a branch and eating a banana next to a magical monkey might cure my cancer, I would have replied, "I'm in! Where can I sign up?"

As odd as I thought this whole spiritual bath and prayer ritual seemed, the fact that Janet had predicted my cancer absolutely terrified me. I followed her advice to a T for my next bath. Precisely as instructed.

I waited until Will left for the office so that I could focus without interruption. Only after the coast was clear and the house was empty did I prepare myself.

I had ordered some white sage from Amazon because, this being a Native American shaman bath, burning some spiritual sage seemed like a suitable idea. As if I knew anything about how to do this, but I guessed my intention was powerful enough.

I cleared a sacred space using my writing desk as an altar, where I carefully arranged my bible, a painting of an angel, and a prayer card of Jesus. I lit a chakra candle along with some yoga incense and burned the sage. I had basically created a custom version of Burning Man in my bedroom.

I pulled up a chair and sat down, trying to calm my mind and enter a deep state of prayer. It took several minutes. I was worried that Will was going to come home and walk into the bedroom, having forgotten his jacket, and then wonder why it smelled like a hippie haven. What nutcase, surrounded by sage smoke, had replaced his wife?

After a few quiet, uninterrupted minutes of focusing on my breath, I was able to push aside all the distracting thoughts of how awkward this all seemed and entered a meditative state. It was time for the first part of Janet's forgiveness prayer ritual.

Janet had explained how a lifetime of feelings of resentment, bitterness, pain, and self-pity, built up inside the heart over the years, can eat away at the spirit like a slowly spreading cancer. It turns out she was right about that, quite literally.

I HOPE THIS HELPS

Find a quiet space with few distractions where you can sit or lie down comfortably and get situated, calm and ready. Call upon God, Jehovah, Allah, Buddha, Sylvia, Dan (for my atheist friends), or someone else. Whoever you ultimately call upon, it should be your version of a higher being. Ask for help to find the powerful energy from within (a.k.a. your higher self). Ask that your desire to put aside all bitterness, wrath, anger, misery and suffering please be granted. You should say this prayer out loud.

Today you wish to truly forgive, once and for all, and to release the malice from deep inside so that you can finally be free. Pray for true forgiveness that will produce a heart that's tender and calm. You are asking for help to choose forgiveness, especially in light of all that you have been forgiven for.

"For if you forgive others their trespasses, your heavenly Father will also forgive you, but if you do not forgive others their trespasses, neither will your Father forgive your trespasses." (Matthew 6:14-15)

I opened by reading the Prayer to St. Francis of Assisi, which hangs as a painting inside of my home. Only after this day did I seem to gain a much deeper connection with it.

Prayer of St. Francis

Lord, make me an instrument of your peace;
where there is hatred, let me sow love;
where there is injury, pardon;
where there is doubt, faith;
where there is despair, hope;
where there is darkness, light;
and where there is sadness, joy;

O Divine Master,
grant that I may not so much seek
to be consoled, as to console;
to be understood, as to understand;
to be loved, as to love;
For it is in giving that we receive;
it is in pardoning that we are pardoned;
and it is in dying that we are born to eternal life.

Amen.

Now is the time when I want you to go as far back in your life as you can remember. Begin to walk through past memories, year by year, allowing anything that comes to your mind to simply enter without judgment.

Do not question it. Just trust that it has appeared for good reason and allow it. Observe it, and once you feel ready to release and forgive this offense, person, grievance, or memory, you may say aloud that you forgive this. Ask that you may hand this over as something you are no longer willing to carry in your heart. When you ask, set your intentions and truly mean this.

Take however long you need going back throughout your entire life, memory by memory. After you have forgiven everyone you feel you need to, now take a moment to forgive yourself.

Remember the many times you have required forgiveness – not so you will live in self-condemnation, but rather so you remain humbly aware of your obligation to extend forgiveness to others as freely as you now are asking to receive it.

Then, let go. Visualize yourself packaging up all the memories you just released into a box, wrapping it up, carefully placing it at your feet. Next, turn and walk away. Don't worry. Someone else is there, ready to carry this package away for you. They know how to process it all for the greater good. This is something you no longer need to worry about. This is no longer your concern because you are now fully free.

Take a few deep cleansing breaths and focus on how you feel inside. A new awareness should prompt a heart full of compassion, kindness, humility, unconditional love, and patience. You should have now released others, and in forgiving them, you, too, have also been forgiven.

Pray that you prevent any root of bitterness from ever springing up inside again. That, when it happens again, you may now recognize this for what it is, and that you will instantly and effortlessly be able to free yourself from those thoughts.

Pray that above all else you now choose to see from a place of unconditional love, which binds everything together in perfect harmony.

Ask that your heart be healed with grace and that, from today forward, you be compelled to let peace rule your mind, body, and spirit.

Acknowledge all the work that you have just done here today, and finally, offer up a moment of thanks and gratitude.

•••

To prepare the cleansing bath, fill your tub with warm, not hot, water. Add ¾ cup of raw apple cider vinegar, sprinkle in 1½ cups of sea salt, and 1½ cups of baking soda. If you like, you may add some essential oil for aromatherapy and to offset the scent of apple cider vinegar. Stir the water. Soak for 20 minutes. Turn on the shower and rinse with or without soap.

As you soak in the salt bath, set an intention of removing all negative energy. This includes energy that has been shared with you by others and energy that you have brought on yourself.

•••

I followed Janet's forgiveness prayer directions exactly as explained above. The early part of my life was relatively easy to go through. It was the last decade that seemed to carry the brunt of the burden. When I arrived at the point where I needed to forgive the people who had caused so much pain and suffering for my family and me, I was overwhelmed with emotion, crying through that uncomfortable part of my prayer.

It was very therapeutic and cathartic. I don't have a therapist. I equate what happened that morning to a powerful mental and spiritual breakthrough, achieved not with the cost of hiring a professional but through my DIY self-care ritual. You could say I had an intervention of the soul through powerful spiritual awakening.

I believe it worked for me because I took it very seriously. If you decide to try this for yourself, please be sure to do the same. If you think you need help from a professional, go that route instead. The point is, do this hard work. Consider it a necessary step in your healing process. After years of failing to effectively let go of all the pain I had carried with me from before that day, I finally let it all go.

I visualized cutting the cords from my belly one last time and instead replaced the black mass with a cleansing white light illuminating from my stomach, shining out of my entire body from head to toe, filling my entire aura with clean and clear light. It was bright and rose far above the top of my head, out through my eyes, my fingertips, and the soles of my feet.

When I came out from my prayer and finally opened my eyes, I noticed that the air around me felt lighter. The room appeared brighter, and I could breathe deeply. The energy in my room had shifted, and I could sense this. The mass was gone.

Now it was time for the next step of the process. I needed to take a spiritual cleansing bath. I carried the incense, candle, and burning sage into the bathroom. As I ran the bathwater, I added the ingredients and set my intentions over the bathtub. I asked that this wash away the last of any remnants needed to fully cleanse my body from cancer, both the form of soul cancer and my now physical colorectal cancer.

The entire prayer and bath process took several hours to complete. Thankfully nobody came home to interrupt or catch me looking like a crazy loon. I am certain that if they had they would have questioned whether my cancer diagnosis had finally pushed me over the deep end, falling far from sanity, tipping the scales of reason to the point of no return.

I don't know why this day was finally the one that made such a drastic difference for me inside. All I can tell you is that, despite my feeling rather silly while doing the work, it accomplished the intended effect.

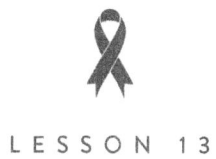

LESSON 13

GET IN TOUCH WITH YOUR SOUL

Life can change in many ways when you or a loved one develops cancer. I found myself turning to my spiritual side to try to cope. I also began to question my own faith.

Why am I here? What is the meaning of life? What is the purpose? Why is life so hard for so many around the world? Why do bad things happen to good people? Why would God allow me to fall in love with my husband and bless us with bringing four beloved children into the world, only to cause us all to suffer should I not survive cancer? How could God, who is supposed to be only made up of good, be so cruel? Does everything truly happen for a reason?

This reaction is quite normal among the many cancer patients and survivors I know. You make an effort to try to reorient your life during a time of crisis. This is a commonly shared experience, and it is important to remember that you're not alone at this time— many people have taken this spiritual journey before you.

Spirituality is a vast subject. Spirituality touches on everything about the world around us, from the explanations we seek for the creation of the universe and our purpose in life to our connection to a higher power behind all these things.

Whether you identify as a religious person of faith, a skeptic, or something in between, the concepts of spirituality, religion, and morality affect us all. It influences the values, laws, and beliefs that govern us and the way we behave, treat one another, and interact with society.

Everyone has a spiritual self. Practicing spirituality, for me, is something that encourages you to feel - in your body and your emotions - a deeper sense of being. It is an excellent way to build on those healing warm and fuzzy feelings we've talked so much about. It helps boost your immune system and is good for you. In addition to helping increase positive emotions and feelings that can help heal, spirituality is a powerful way to find much-needed comfort.

Many have experienced moments when they have felt connected to a deeper meaning or reality. Spirituality is an experience that is much like that of a soothing warm blanket or an invisible wave that washes over you, leaving a tremendous sense of peace and grace. You can feel an out-of-body sensation separate from your five senses, a sixth sense, and one that is experienced deeply from within.

You have likely felt this too. It's a sensation of calmness. Like when you embrace and hug someone that you deeply love, lose yourself in space and time gazing up at the stars and moon, or happen to catch the perfect sunrise or sunset.

I believe that at our core we are all spiritual beings, made up of energy. I believe we are all here having a temporary human experience inside of our body and in what we call life. I also believe in life after death. I believe that our spiritual energy existed before we were born and will continue to do so after our physical body dies.

If my referencing your spiritual self still makes you cringe, then you can go ahead and call it a deep, peaceful energy that flows through us all. One that is experienced through feeling intense emotion and physical sensation. Some call this "prana'. Others call it "chi." What you call it matters less than how you connect with it.

The topic is an incredibly delicate subject for many, and for this reason, I want to tread lightly. For some, what I say will hit close to home, but for others, I fully understand this can cause many to abruptly shut down. Let me be clear that I am not here to preach, persuade or try to convince you about my personal spiritual beliefs.

I will continue to share several examples of how I grew a stronger connection to my spiritual self through my experience with cancer, as this is a book about my personal story; but I fully expect that every person reading this will have their own unique interpretation of what it means for them, and their personal interpretation may be very different from that of my own.

My spiritual self surpasses my religious beliefs. Spirit is connected with your life force and directly related to your purpose in life. Religion is just one of many ways I connect to spirituality. Regardless of your religious affiliation, or lack thereof, deepening a connection to your spiritual self is a practice that is open to all.

Spiritual moments can happen at any time, anywhere, and to anyone—for example, when you feel close to nature, look into the eyes of a loved one, enter a house of worship or sense the presence of a higher power.

I've quoted the bible and shared that I was raised as a Christian. I am married to a Catholic and have family members and friends of all different religious denominations, backgrounds, and beliefs.

My favorite college courses were Anthropology and Religious Studies. I believe all humans are born with the instinct to explore and we spend much of our lives seeking answers to our very existence. It was in the classroom and through international travel that I discovered I believe so much more than what I was exposed to in my home and church.

I have always been intrigued to develop a greater understanding of the evolution of mankind and to study the lifestyle differences between cultures and behavioral patterns. How that is all tied to cultural constructs, history, philosophy, ethics, and so forth.

I personally opt to pull from everything that I have learned and that has resonated in my soul. That is a vast compilation of the teachings from my Christian upbringing as well as Buddhism, Confucianism, Islam, Judaism, Hinduism, Sikhism, Indigenous American Religions, and many more.

I believe all these different beliefs share many common core values and offer the experience of coming together to worship as a means to connect with others. This is where I believe organized religion gets it right.

Where it fails us, however, is the moment it starts to divide and separate us from one another. So much about our modern lifestyle has us living individually focused. We live independently and have sadly come to view ourselves as separate from others.

Spirituality tells us to do the exact opposite. It brings us all together. It reminds us that we are all intimately connected to one another, made up of the same spiritual energy, and come from the source. Spirituality is all about universal love. The deepest love there is. It is finding total peace with everything and everyone.

The God I have come to know is all-loving. The moment we place conditions upon that love is when it becomes irrelevant to me; conditions such as which religion we identify with, which name we call God, which house we worship in, which scripture we read. Spirituality is bigger than organized religion. It is open to all, offering us a deep connection to one another as a powerful shared human experience.

For me, God is in all things and part of all people. God loves you no matter who you are or where you are from. God is always gentle, kind, humble, meek, and patient. God is compassionate.

God loves unconditionally. No conditions are ever placed on us in order to receive or be deemed worthy of this love. There's no need to repent or follow an established set of rules that people have created from their interpretation of scripture.

The God I know doesn't punish. Nor does God allow for some to burn in eternal damnation while sparing the lives of others. God loves not only some, but all of us. Regardless of who you are, the language you speak, your race, nationality, your religion, or who you love. There simply are no conditions on God's love. Love is love. Period.

God is the ultimate form of love. A miraculous source of energy we can all sense and feel inside. We all experience that love, regardless of how we ultimately connect with this source through our spiritual self. I believe that part of my physical healing was due to this connection to deeper and higher energy.

I believe in the power of prayer. I believe that the many who prayed for me, setting their minds and intentions for my healing, made a difference in my recovery. I had Catholic parishioners, Christian bible study partners, dear Muslim friends, and even atheists forest-bathing in nature sending me their highest healing vibes. No one was more powerful than the other. Their belief that there is a higher power that could help me heal was all I needed to receive it. I gratefully welcomed prayer in every form it came from.

Whatever your personal spiritual beliefs are, remember that spirituality is a dimension of your life that can be developed and strengthened. I encourage everyone to get to know their spiritual self.

I Hope This Helps

Get outside and into nature. I walk or run at least four days a week outdoors. I use this time to listen to a book, podcast, or calming music, but I also often opt to quiet my mind and simply observe everything around me. Take it all in. Nature brings such a sense of peace, gratitude, and higher connection. I feel very connected to God when alone in this space. Inspirational thoughts flow freely to my mind when I'm outdoors. I feel most present while enjoying the sights of the rolling hillside, the smell of fresh rain, the sound of leaves rustling in the wind, and the feeling of blades of grass beneath my bare feet.

Meditate. It is easy to access guided meditation from podcasts, apps, and many of the latest streaming services. I feel more peaceful after listening to meditations and playlists of healing sounds and music. I fall asleep to this and often begin my morning to favorites such as Jai-Jagdeesh's Aad Guray Nameh. Aad Guray Nameh is a very powerful mantra used for protection, to gain clarity, and to receive guidance from one's highest Self. This mantra helps to create a protective field of energy around the person chanting, attracting abundance to help them live out their destiny. Namaste.

Try breathing exercises. Apps like Calm are an excellent resource for practicing deep breaths. You can do this on your own and schedule time to take breaths several times a day. Take a minute to place all thoughts and activities aside and take ten deep inhalations and exhalations. Notice how your body moves and feels as your diaphragm rises and falls with every breath.

Practice visualization and imagery. I often used the practice of mental imagery and imagination to take myself away from what I saw or felt in the present moment, opting to focus instead on how I wanted to feel and what I wanted to see. Whether it was escaping chemotherapy to visit my happy place at my dream home, hosting a retreat at Sámara Sueños in Costa Rica; or experiencing milestone moments with my family five, ten, and twenty years out. This can help trick the mind to stop thinking or feeling in the present moment. Daydreaming is a powerful practice. Rather than letting your head run wild, you can take control to see, feel, taste, and fully immerse yourself in another experience entirely. Ideally one that calms you, reduces blood pressure and heart rate, and boosts the immune response, offering you hope while manifesting future-focused wishes.

Read spiritual work. These can range from the Holy Bible to the Holy Quran to The Dao De Jing; really, any faith-based scripture. You may even use more recently published work like *A Course in Miracles* by Helen Schucman or *Dying to Be Me* by Anita Moorjani. Delving into sacred words can put you in touch with ancient traditions and teachings and the wisdom of influencers and thought provokers and offer you a sense of connection with the divine. Recently published books on spirituality can bring you equally reflective insights like those that have inspired many through the test of time.

Pray. If prayer is something you like to practice, set aside time each day and pray. I recited the Lord's Prayer and the Prayer of St. Francis. Among many other bible scriptures and bible studies, I often read Psalm 91 during my season with cancer. Prayer can offer a sense of comfort and stability. As I've said before, I wholeheartedly believe that the power of prayer indeed works miracles—prayers from others and that of your own. I find mine are always answered and tend to work best when I ask from a place of how I may serve or how I can use this for good, rather than pleading for what I want but don't currently have.

Take a retreat. Visit historical and spiritual spaces, get out into nature, rock out at a concert, or take a trip to a place that inspires you. I am a big fan of retreats. I joined two charitable cancer groups that offer retreats specifically for cancer patients and survivors; they helped me take time away from my usual family responsibilities to get in touch with others who could closely relate to living with cancer. Taking a retreat may help you cultivate a sense of peace and a deeper connection to yourself and the world.

Seek the help of others. Spiritual support is widely accessible, and you might begin with opening a dialogue with a member of the clergy or a spiritual life coach. Many spiritual advisors are trained to talk about the major questions of life, death, and existence. They can also help you create a legacy in your life and find your purpose. Some advisors are religion-based, but many work with people from every faith and background, including those with no religious affiliation. You can also join groups for meditation, prayer, and support. My best advice is to trust your instinct and be selective until you find a spiritual support system with others that you are comfortable with.

Keep a journal. Writing in a private journal to express your feelings, thoughts, and memories can be a wonderful way to connect with your spiritual self. I obviously love to write and believe doing so can contribute to a process of self-discovery and development. I have received a lot of valuable insights and spiritual epiphanies through my personal daily writing practice. Many came to me while writing this book.

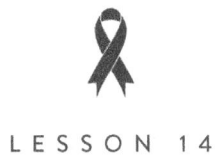

LESSON 14

SURROUND YOURSELF WITH LOVE

Telling family members that I had cancer was the most difficult conversation I have ever had to hold. My mom and stepdad were there with me when I first received the diagnosis, but I had to inform my husband and the rest of my entire family about what had just happened. Breaking this kind of devastating news to those you love is just as tough as it is receiving it for yourself. Sharing with my husband and children was by far the hardest part.

They say that nobody fights alone. When it comes to catastrophic illness or traumatic life-altering experiences, the repercussions hit hard and are felt by all family members. A life crisis often requires changes for more than the person being directly impacted.

There is no convenient age to receive a cancer diagnosis, but young adults, parents in particular, have to juggle a unique set of circumstances. Life doesn't stop after your cancer diagnosis. Bills still need to be paid, kids need help with homework, errands need to be run, meals must be prepared; there are never-ending responsibilities that caring for a family entails.

My goal with this next section of the book is to offer a fearless appraisal of what it means to be uncertain about your future - all while juggling the intensity of family life. I hope to teach you how to best navigate the chaos of parenting while dealing with catastrophic illness and crisis.

THE MOTHER OF ALL FIGHTS

•••

When Will and I said our vows, "For better or worse, till death do us part," neither one of us realized how much this promise would be tested in our marriage. Looking back over our 17 years in a relationship together, we have weathered some substantial life storms, including many most marriages will never face after a lifetime together.

Our loyalty and love for one another is bonded and has been proven time and again. Living with me as your other half is what I describe as being anything but easy. Tolerating me under extreme pressure is even more daunting a task; I have a reputation for not coping well under high stress.

Will deserves a medal for his patience and putting up with me and all the crazy that comes with my total package. I often tell him how grateful I am to have him by my side. Every day I am reminded of how I can hardly live without him.

As in most marriages, we have had seasons of highs and lows. There were years in which our marriage was greatly tested and strained. I genuinely believe that it was persevering through the hardest times, especially my cancer, that brought us closer together.

Surviving all that we have is proof that I indeed married my forever soulmate. Marriage requires never-ending work and intentional effort. Four children, lawsuits, intense financial struggle, and catastrophic sickness were an awful lot to navigate through. Understandably, they tested our limits.

Will and I often joke that, from the lowest of low points we reached together, the only option we had was to move onward and upward. On the bright side, we are both eager for the days where our greatest worries revolve around small problems, like raising four hungry and hormonal teenagers, saving for college tuition (x4), and dealing with what I would describe as the normal challenges most face. After what we have conquered together thus far, much of the stuff that others may tend to perceive as big problems in their grand scheme of life sounds like a walk in the park and smooth sailing to us.

I told Will just earlier this morning that this is the first time in too long that we can recount that life seems peaceful and relatively easy. Today we are living our version of happily ever after, still fresh off my recent remission status, praying that we can continue to feel gratitude well into old age over my recovering health and the many freedoms that it brings for our entire family.

We wake up every morning full of thanks but also aware that what feels like solid ground is, in fact, ever-changing and always unstable—as is life. It is up to us to concentrate on protecting our relationship and the solid foundation we have built so that when the next storm does blow through, we can weather whatever comes our way.

I admit that, ever since wrapping cancer treatment, it has been a daily challenge to not fear that, if I allow myself to feel too comfortable or enjoy the moment, it will be abruptly stolen away. It's as though I'm always waiting for the next ball to drop again at any given moment. Post-traumatic stress and high anxiety are common experiences many cancer survivors battle. Will is thankfully my solid rock when I feel shaken. He keeps me standing firm in faith and has a way of keeping me centered amidst the times when I allow my doubts and fears to start to creep in and get the best of me.

He is the one reminding me that it is perfectly okay, in fact, very important, that I learn to embrace and lean into the new and unusual sense of comfort and peace we have today. Commit myself to feeling and even celebrating it so that we can expect to experience more of it. Don't overthink it, but simply appreciate the grace this day brings. Relish in the wonderful smooth sailing without worrying so much about whatever our next storm will bring. We'll stay the course and will always have each other when that time comes.

I cannot imagine going through life without Will. He is my greatest love, my best friend, and my true one-and-only soul mate. I couldn't have asked for a more dedicated, loving husband and father to our children, and I have so much admiration for all he does to keep this family thriving.

All I hope for is for us to simply experience ease, peace, joy, health, and the gift to continue to be able to embrace our second chance, after all we just survived.

Will was as terrified by my diagnosis as I was. We both felt anxious, helpless, and lost about what to do. We were very much distraught over what this could mean for our children. He was our solid rock, putting on a brave face for the kids and me, but I could see the deep fear he carried within when I looked into his eyes. He had to be the strong one; even on days he felt weary. Relationships often tend to work like an ebb and flow or yin and yang. When one person falls, the other will compensate by rising to the occasion. Will stepped up to help us face this rough season.

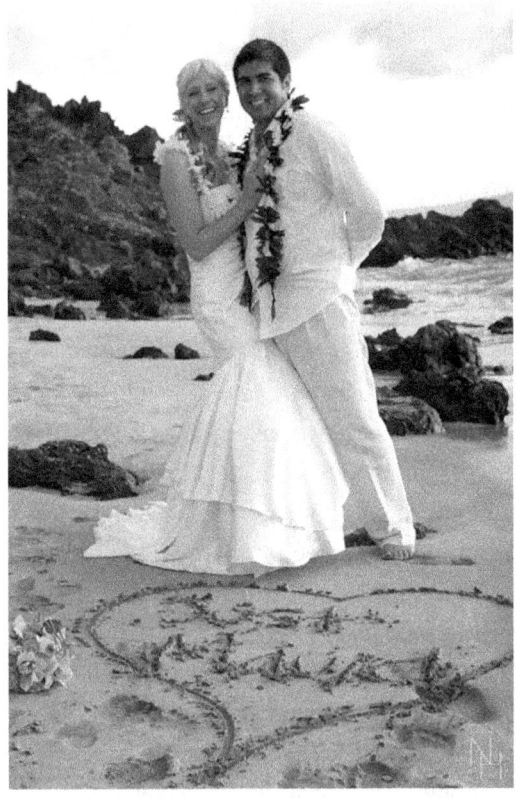

For better or worse; till death do us part.

∙ ∙ ∙

As parents, we try our best to teach our children all about life, but they are often the ones teaching us what life is all about. I struggled with not wanting to take away my kids' sense of normalcy, security, and joy by introducing my traumatic disease into their world.

I desperately wanted to shield my children from having to deal with cancer and the pain it would no doubt introduce them to. I viewed cancer as a big bad beast, here to steal away some of their childhood innocence and joy. I wanted to protect them. I knew full well how much the hurt of all that was to come would inevitably change them.

I hated that this was now going to become a part of their childhood story and a problem they, too, would have to learn to live and cope with directly. I also know that children have no filter and are likely going to ask the hardest questions, the ones that everyone else I broke the news to would be too polite to bring up.

The questions I myself hadn't been comfortable enough to fully digest yet, with answers they had every right to know. Questions like, "Are you going to die, Mommy?" were inevitable. I needed to be incredibly careful in how I responded to that, mindful about what information I shared and how I presented answers to them. Those words could come back to take on a deeper meaning for them someday in the future—the worst-case scenario. I decided that complete transparency and honesty were key when telling the children about my cancer.

Will and I were going to hold the conversations with our kids together, and we waited a good week before finally mustering up the courage we both needed to sit down and talk with them.

I have never been more terrified to talk about a hard thing in all of my life. This was hands down the most difficult of all the family conversations that I had to hold. There is no way to properly prepare anyone for this; but it is something that you have to do, like it or not, given the circumstances.

My youngest boys were still at an age when I knew the term cancer wouldn't resonate. Liam was only four years old, and Taylor was just seven at the time. My twins, however, Cristian and Sienna, were ten, and telling them meant having a very different conversation. Will and I decided it ought to be broken into separate talks. We knew the twins would both have a lot of questions, and we wanted to give them our full, undivided, parent-to-child attention.

Breaking the news caused confusion, fear, and heartbreak. All of the kids were understandably very upset. This was a sad day in the Soto home, and if you had been a fly on the wall you likely would have been in tears right along with the rest of us. I hope you never have to hold a conversation like this yourself as a parent. But if you do, should this be something you, too, have to face, I will share what I learned from my own experience with my kids to help prepare you.

I didn't want to pretend that everything was going to be okay because I knew they were going to see and experience all that would happen along with me. It was important to be honest. Everything I had read about how to tell your kids you have cancer suggests that telling the truth is better than letting them imagine the worst. I gave them plenty of time to ask as many questions as they needed answers for.

The little ones sensed that something was very wrong, but the initial talk with them was far easier than with my twins. My littlest two boys were both impacted more later, when seeing me actually go through my cancer treatment in real-time, suffering physically in plain sight. That proved to impact each of them immensely. The preparation conversation was less intense as they really could not grasp what this meant.

My youngest, Liam, often still liked to sit on my lap and cuddle or be carried. He needed to be reminded how he now needed to be extra gentle around my cancer boo-boos, avoid touching my chemo port, and in general be gentle with my body. Mommy wasn't going to be able to pick him up as I previously had, even though we both wanted more than ever for this to happen. That was something he and I struggled with adjusting to.

Liam acted out from the changes that watching me get sick caused. This often was worst on days when he could see that I really wasn't feeling well, like times when I was absent and away from home at the hospital for treatment, and during the following chemotherapy infusion days.

It was a result of my not spending nearly as much time with him in the same manner he was accustomed to and, due to his young age, still needed. I wanted to take him to picnics at the park and lay on the floor playing games with him, following our usual morning routine of quality time enjoyed together; but now my days were filled with feeling sick, often needing to rest in bed. This change hurt me as much as it did him.

Just this last Christmas, a little more than a year following my diagnosis, I asked Liam, who was now five years old, what he wanted Santa Claus to bring him. He replied that he only wanted Mommy to be home this time for Christmas, and for me not to keep going back to the hospital again. He wanted my cancer to go away forever and wanted everyone else in the whole world to be healthy too because cancer and COVID were bad.

It goes without saying, this last year clearly made an impression on him at a very young age. Santa brought him an electric scooter for Christmas, and thankfully, the week of Christmas, he also brought Liam the glorious news of Mommy's cancer remission. So sweet Liam got his Christmas wish delivered by Santa early this year. His wish proved how even the youngest children carry the weight from this kind of traumatic experience in more ways than we would ever wish on our beloved children.

My second youngest, Taylor, has always been my affectionate love bug. He wanted to nurse Mommy back to health with plenty of hugs, often sitting beside me and tending to my needs whenever I was sick in bed. He would sometimes get very sad and cry and would share with me how he wished I could play with him in the ways I used to. But he also understood, better than Liam, what was happening to his mom and that my not doing so wasn't by choice. His bright spirit and compassionate care often lifted me up on the days I desperately needed his ray of sunshine, smiles, and cuddles.

I don't believe that my daughter, Sienna, had realized anything was drastically wrong with me, despite knowing about my recent and frequent visits in and out of the hospital over the weeks leading up to our cancer conversation. When we finally sat her down to share the news, we seemed to catch her completely off guard.

Parents are superheroes in the eyes of their children, and the thought of Mom being dangerously sick seemed impossible for her to grasp. I have always been very active and involved in her life and, physically, an example of strength. I've coached her sports teams, led her girl scout troops, and we often played together doing somersaults and handstands in the yard, swinging on the swing set, and jumping on our trampoline. Viewing Mom as someone who was now very sick, with the possibility of dying, was a foreign concept. She was incredibly upset, afraid, and overwhelmed by what her mom having cancer might mean.

Over the course of the coming year, she would also come to take on a lot of my motherly role and responsibility in caring for her brothers. I often joked she was ten years going on 25. She would cuddle the younger boys to sleep, help give them their evening baths, serve them snacks, and kiss and bandage boo-boos, taking care to do so the same exact way Mommy would have if she could have done so herself.

Sienna often very much acted as the mommy for her younger brothers; but she still was a young child herself. I hated watching her have to grow up faster than she should have needed to as a result of my sickness. She did it all with grace. She is one tough girl, a very caring sister, and an incredibly admirable daughter of whom I am so proud.

Her twin brother, Cristian, has always been an old soul, wise beyond his years. He is also our extra-sensitive child. Of all four kids, the news of my cancer seemed to hit him the hardest. He is incredibly intelligent. He knew exactly what cancer meant without us having to explain much to him. The moment the "C" word was shared, he immediately started to cry. He was the one who asked the tough questions that nobody else had the nerve to.

He wanted to know if I was going to die. He wanted to know what "sick" meant and how sick I was going to become. Just typing this now and reliving this memory brings me back to that conversation, and tears.

I had to explain to Cristian that just because I had cancer didn't mean

I would necessarily die from it, but that, yes, death was a possibility. I had to explain there was no way of knowing whether or not I would survive this. I couldn't guarantee that my surgery or chemotherapy would work. I then told him how many people live with terminal cancer for years, and how others are lucky enough for it not to recur. Many with cancer will fully recover in remission and live out the rest of their lives, having restored their health. Unfortunately, I couldn't predict the future for how my body would respond to cancer treatment or if I would ultimately come to survive this.

I explained that I had been diagnosed with an advanced form of cancer at Stage 3, and that was a little disheartening; but many others before me have fully recovered and we should hold onto the hope that I might, too. That was what we all must hope, pray, and wish for.

I made a heartfelt promise to all of my kids that although so much of this is out of our control, they could count on me to do absolutely everything in my power to survive this. I was going to fight for every last breath, every minute, hour, and miraculous day of life. I prayed furiously for perfect health and more time. I wanted nothing more than to be alive, to be here with them as they go through much more of their lives.

I wanted to watch them all grow up. The gift of time was something I'd always appreciated, but in the face of losing what mattered most to me, the many privileges of parenting my kids, the gift of love and being with family, was the most brutal blow my cancer diagnosis landed. I wanted to come out from cancer healed, with the grace of living out the remainder of my life, into old age, with my family. I couldn't promise my kids that this would happen but assured them I was going to fight for this and give absolutely every ounce of my being to do just that.

I also told them how they never needed to worry about these painful and frightening thoughts because no matter what happened to me and with my life, they would always be together and would be taken care of by our family members, no matter what.

Lastly, I explained it was more than okay to get upset and angry, and to feel scared and sad. I reminded them our entire family was all here to help. Will and I asked them to let us know any time they needed someone to talk to. We explained that if they didn't feel comfortable talking to us about this, we would get them another adult who could listen to them and offer them help.

Looking back, I can say this experience affected every single one of my four children deeply and differently. I believe that in many ways we all grew stronger through it and have become closer as a family because of it. That doesn't mean it didn't hurt them during the process. They had to learn to live under the same pressures and constant sense of worry we all felt during the journey.

It was a painful time with some frighteningly close calls that have left deep wounds on us all. Knowing and seeing the ways that this has impacted the kids is possibly the worst part of all.

In the end, my kids showed me how resilient they are. Together, we gained wisdom through every member of our family's personal experience. We gained hard-earned life lessons growing through this as a family.

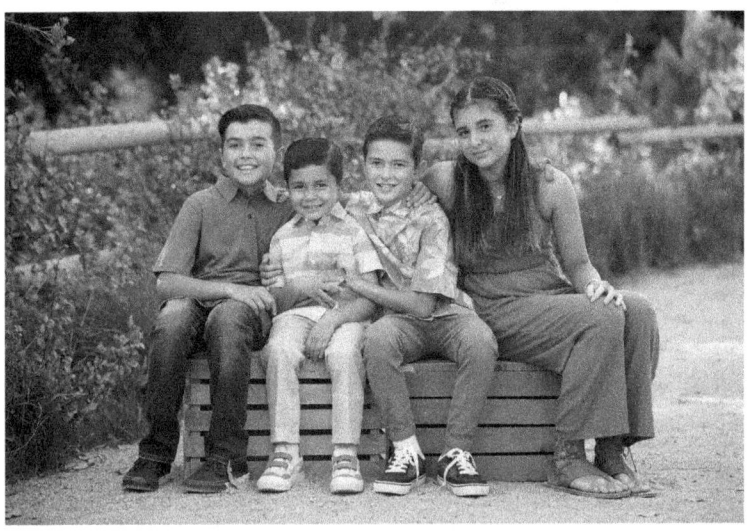

Soto sibling strong. Cristian, Liam, Taylor and Sienna.

• • •

I couldn't continue with having to break the news to my sister, brothers, and in-laws. Things were becoming just too much to tolerate, and I was already hurting enough trying to digest the changes I was experiencing myself. I wanted to focus on being present to help my kids navigate the news and the subsequent life changes we were going through. I let my parents and husband take on the burden of telling the rest of my family members for me.

Cancer affects every person in the entire family, not just the one with cancer or those living under your roof. The people in your life will also feel worried, angry, or afraid. My family members were thankfully all incredibly supportive and ready to drop what was going on in their own lives to rush to our aid at a moment's notice.

My dad tried to remain optimistic, reminding me how strong he thought I was and how he believed I was going to beat this. I could hear in his voice that he was also scared, but he wasn't going to say it. At least he wasn't willing to admit it to me, for my own sake. I don't know what happened after hanging up the phone with my dad on the day I told him I had cancer, but I know that this is a call no parent ever wants to receive from their child. Even if their child is all grown up.

My dad was recently retired and recovering from a knee replacement, but he got into his car with my stepmom, who requested a few weeks off from work, and they hurried to our home. They drove down from Sacramento, arriving a couple of days just before my operation to help with the kids, to help with the move from house to apartment, and to salvage what they could for the kids around the holiday.

My little sister, Stacy, is an elementary school teacher. She drove down immediately following Christmas to also support us, bringing along one of my nieces. The first time she called me after learning about my diagnosis was super emotional. She was in a state of shock and disbelief, and while I tried to play the big sister role and console her by telling her I was going to be just fine and was managing it all rather well, she couldn't help starting to cry on the other end of the phone; the next thing I knew we were both in tears together.

I was in the car line waiting to pick up my kids from school and had to hang up because I started to lose my own ability to hold it together. I didn't want the kids to get into the car and find their mom crying uncontrollably. My sister checked in with me often and sent me a lot of care packages, always there cheering me on during my entire fight with cancer.

My sister and my mom's twin sister, Aunt Lynne, had both come down to help right after Christmas. My aunt came just as much to support my mom and to help her care for my stepdad so that she could remain by my side. My aunt also worked tirelessly helping care for the kids and me. Will's family, his mom, sister and brother and their families, also provided tremendous support. Without help from so many of my family members, we never would have been able to get through moving out of our house and into the apartment.

On the bright side, they were all way more organized than I was and packed up our entire home more efficiently than I would have done on my own. It was like an episode of hoarders going through seven years' and six people's worth of accumulated stuff. So much unnecessary junk. Especially since we had just gone through the season of having babies and young children, which tends to require accumulating a lot of kiddie gadgets and gizmos.

Thankfully, they packed us up and talked me into thinning out our family's belongings and minimizing the mounds of unnecessary stuff we no longer needed. We could start fresh, clean, and clear after our big move.

We were downsizing from a five-bedroom home into a tiny short-term rental apartment, so we had to prioritize keeping only what we needed and loved. We had a small storage unit and sold whatever wouldn't fit. The move and many items we sold helped to pay off the first medical bills nearing $10,000, and we applied the rest toward our mountain of debt and effort to save for the future.

The move was supposed to feel like a step toward our dream of relocating to Costa Rica and getting our lives on track and regaining control over our finances; but now the move was overshadowed by my disease and no longer carried the sense of adventure we had originally hoped to achieve from it.

Instead, it felt like a part of the unraveling firestorm that had literally engulfed us in flames, burning down the foundation of our former dream home, leaving us with nothing but ashes and memories of our lost dreams—left only with an uncertain future to look to.

Sometimes, this kind of total loss is absolutely necessary. In order to fully release what no longer serves you, you must destroy every lasting remnant of the old, down to the very last splinter, leaving anything unnecessary behind. Only then can one begin to rebuild a newer, better, and more solid foundation for the future. I would indeed eventually come to create a masterful work of art out of the ashes of trauma. It literally took feeling like we had lost it all before the explosive and transformative life growth could happen.

The timing of the move was horrendous but cleaning out our belongings was necessary and actually proved to serve us well in the long run. We were forced to finally declutter our life during a state of utter chaos. Lightening the load of belongings was actually very freeing.

To thank the ladies in my life, one afternoon I treated them all to high tea as a way of showing my gratitude for everything they had done to support us during those difficult weeks of transition.

My stepmom and sister had to return home and get back to work before the new year, but my dad and aunt stayed to help all the way through the entire holiday season, and, after our move, through the first few weeks of 2020. Having them there to help was the greatest gift, and to this day I am still overcome with tremendous gratitude to have been surrounded with so much love and support.

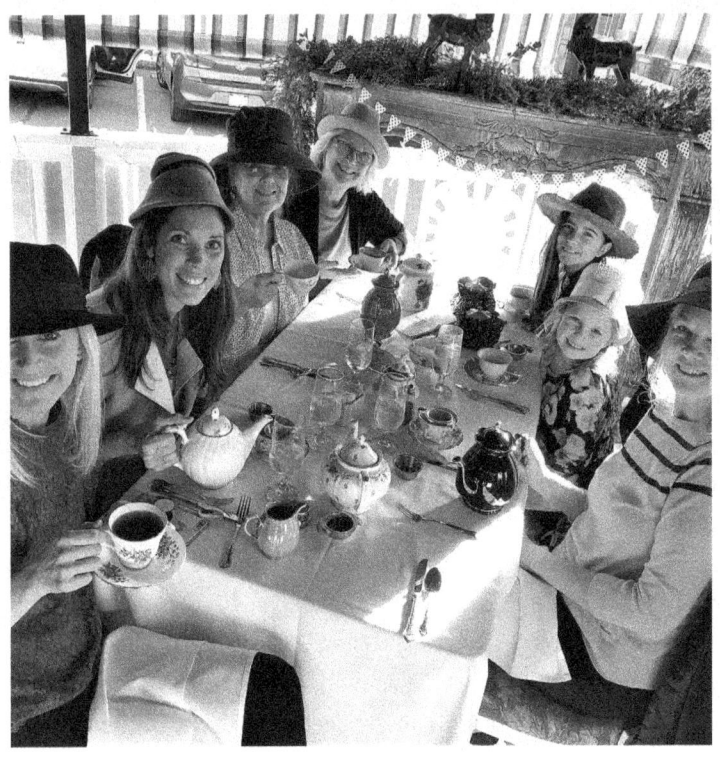

An afternoon tea party to thank the ladies I love most.
Me, Stacy, Aunt Lynne, Mom, Sienna, Madeleine and my stepmom, Irene.

• • •

Cancer is hard on everyone. Most especially the people who love and care for you. The changes can take a toll on your family members. Those caring for you can become run down and get tired from all the stress. Be careful to check in often and ask how they are coping.

I was the patient, but what I learned was how difficult my being sick also was for my husband, parents, and children. They were in the entire ordeal with me, day in and day out. We all had days where it just felt like too much.

Everyone is going to need to find balance in their life and ways to cope when the going gets too heavy. Be sure to allow plenty of time to take care of yourself and your many life responsibilities. Prioritize time to rest, to just enjoy the company of family and friends, or to do your favorite hobbies.

The exact same advice can be said for your caregivers. They, too, will need to sort through their emotions and the challenges of living with your having cancer. Be sure to schedule time for them to have needed breaks. Remember, nobody fights alone. Together, you will learn and grow and may even come to discover that this brings you closer.

•••

A common theme of most moms I know is that it feels there's always more to do than time to do it. I was slowed down by my cancer, but all of my to-dos still existed. I had to learn to do something that didn't come very naturally to me. I had to learn how to ask for and receive help from others.

I have always been eager to volunteer and lend a helping hand. I prided myself as being a woman of service, often offering my time and resources to school, sports associations, church, and other community resources. I've coached countless youth athletic teams, regularly volunteered at food pantries and animal shelters, delivered casseroles and meals to families following a new baby or health crisis, and tried to give back in every way possible for the greater good. I was a professional giver, always eager to care for others in times of need.

I was also the primary caretaker of my own household. I kissed boo-boos and generated clever solutions for all my family's most distressing and seemingly insurmountable problems. I had supermom powers and could practically fix every problem that my kids brought to me. Until, one day, I woke up facing a monstrous beast of an obstacle that even I couldn't make go away or find a quick fix to solve. I had no answer, nor did I have a way out of the predicament my family was suddenly facing. The only solution was to ask for help.

Receiving help was an entirely foreign concept to me, therefore not my strong point. I associated asking for help with admitting defeat or showing a sign of weakness. Looking back, I now see how ludicrous and backward my thinking was at the time, but this was honestly how I felt.

It was as though overnight I went from supporting my favorite charitable causes to becoming a charity case myself. I didn't want others to take pity on my family and me. I hated being the topic of conversation in our social circles and the attention that accompanied my new title transition from "Supermom" to "Cancer-mom."

The negative circumstances my family and I now found ourselves surrounded by were not something I embraced or felt comfortable allowing others an insider's perspective on. This was my personal problem and my very own private business. I also knew that we had no other option than to accept as much help as we could find if we wanted to hold onto any chance of surviving this crisis.

I sat down in the kitchen one morning alongside my mom and Will, having come to realize how much they were each scrambling in an effort to tackle my many usual roles and responsibilities, all while caring for me in a now full-time capacity. We desperately needed emergency aid.

Their suggestion that I ask for assistance made me cringe in utter discomfort, and I seriously struggled over it. This was a new and awkward position to be in, but I needed to get over my ego and swallow my pride.

They say that giving to others is a selfish act because you are really giving yourself all the joy that doing so brings you. Helping others, without expecting anything in return, is what self-worth is really all about. It offers a sense of purpose and meaning to life. It is human nature to want to help someone.

It's no wonder that extending care and compassion to someone in need feels like such a natural response. It's also why accepting help is our next topic to cover as a necessary step in recovery.

There really is no better feeling than offering help, and I believe that most people can, and will, do some remarkable things to assist you in your greatest hour of need. This can only happen, of course, after you get out of your own way and become open and willing to accept it.

That was a life lesson I was practically forced into mastering overnight. After everything that had happened, Will had encouraged me to reach out to friends and share the news of my diagnosis, but I didn't want to burden friends by sharing my sob story about our family's new problems.

I reluctantly agreed, but only after Will and my mom pointed out the desperate situation that was now surrounding our family due to my sudden health predicament. Our circumstances were so dire that I doubt we would have gotten through another week without relying on the support of those willing to come to our rescue.

After several days of contemplating how best to go about sharing the news, I decided that doing so over social media seemed like the easiest plan. I could share all the gory details in one big announcement. It would be like ripping off a band-aid. I also liked that I could hide behind the safety of my computer screen while not having to see or hear other people's reactions after they learned about my having cancer.

I couldn't bear the thought of having to retell the story and relive the entire experience over and over again. One fell swoop in the form of a Facebook post would do the trick. You've already seen exactly what I shared in that post itself, but what you don't know is what happened after I shared it. I posted my announcement and immediately responses started to trickle in from concerned friends asking how they could help.

I was still processing the diagnosis myself at the time and didn't want any part in the many incoming conversations. Talking about it with my own family was difficult enough. Thankfully, my mom and a couple of friends rose to the occasion and took leadership over the task of generating a list of ways to best offer us support.

They first organized shifts of volunteers to help us with our house move. Some came to our home and helped pack our belongings into moving boxes. Others brought their trucks and did manual labor and heavy lifting of furniture out of our house and over to our apartment, which was inconveniently located on the second floor of a building without an elevator. Some helped us unpack every room, from our kitchen to the kids' new bedrooms, all working together to make our temporary home as cozy and functional as possible. We could never have gotten through that major move without everyone's assistance.

I HOPE THIS HELPS

Just like what you put into your body, it's time to get picky about who you spend your time with. If we are all energy, then you need to surround yourself with people who boost that energy, not drain it. Take some time to list all the people who are currently in your life and decide what they are bringing to it. Are they positive? Are they unnecessarily negative? Notice how people show up. And for the time being, while you're healing, get really selective on who you allow into your presence. If you can't avoid Negative Nellies altogether, then limit your time in their company or schedule in a way that allows you to recoup any lost energy from their visits. Collect a cancer crew that you know is creating a healing environment and keep it close, as if your life depends on it, because it does!

PART V

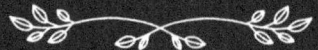

The Student Becomes
the Teacher

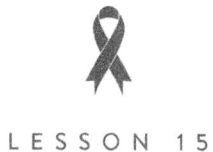

LESSON 15

Become a Master in Handling Setbacks

As Dr. Parker forewarned, during my chemotherapy not once, but twice I was deemed too sick to continue treatment. My lab results, taken prior to each chemotherapy session, proved that the chemotherapy was indeed working powerfully, so effectively obliterating cancer cells that I had reached a point where it was no longer safe to continue with my next infusion. I was dangerously low in white blood count and deemed too fragile to withstand treatment for fear of my being unable to tolerate pushing my body any further. It could be too much.

Dr. Parker had warned me that this was likely going to happen before we even began treatment. He'd covered how many of the chemotherapy patients on my regimen are not able to finish all twelve rounds due to it being far too potent for them to tolerate. Despite knowing this was always a possibility, that didn't make it any less exasperating when I received the news. I felt devastated, helpless, fragile, weak, and incapable. I felt like I was starting to fail, and that the cancer was maybe winning.

It was now late April, and while I was well into working my way through more than half of my chemotherapy infusions, I was beginning to lose my inner fight to go on. With the sudden explosion of the coronavirus pandemic in the months before, the entire world was now living with a great deal of fear, uncertainty, and anxiety. As a cancer patient, those feelings were certainly heightened, making an already very difficult time only that much more challenging to cope with.

I was already facing the shock of cancer and the many trials and tribulations that accompanied it. On top of all that, learning that people with cancer were at a much higher risk of severe illness from COVID-19, because treatment made them more vulnerable to complications, was distressing.

I was hearing stories from cancer patients who were unable to have the lifesaving surgeries they required because hospitals were overrun with coronavirus patients. Access to needed cancer treatment was being delayed for many, and for some, it was no longer an option.

I was so grateful to have been able to complete my operation and to have begun receiving chemotherapy treatment before things fell apart. I felt I had somehow managed to dodge a bullet just in the nick of time. That said, going to the hospital for ongoing treatment during the pandemic was nerve-rattling. My frequent trips to a place where coronavirus posed a great threat to cancer patients were unsettling. And yet, despite feeling so frightened, I had to take the risk and continue to show up for my chemotherapy infusions, lab work, and the many doctors' appointments related to treatment. I was terrified by the virus and what it might mean with my having cancer. I had to continue with my treatment, nevertheless, knowing full well that if I did not it could be a matter of my own survival.

To make matters worse, not being able to have family members accompany me during this time, to provide needed moral support, made the entire experience that much more difficult and lonelier than it already was. This was a point in my cancer story where I was starting to struggle most. Spending so much time isolated and alone during treatment forced me more than before to learn how to become incredibly close with my inner thoughts and deeply connected to my body and self.

As I neared the final rounds of chemotherapy, when interruptions in my cancer treatment happened, it would take several days for the setback to settle in. I would eventually decide to accept it as a gift for much-needed rest, taking advantage of it by making the most of my respite. I used the extra weeks forced by the delay of ongoing treatment to enjoy the freedom this granted, the time to do the many things I often wanted to do, but couldn't, because I was too sick, weak, or constantly tied up at the hospital. I played more with my kids and enjoyed the quality family time through every one of the disruptions my treatment plan required.

I would remind myself that, while this might first appear to be a setback, it was exactly what I really needed, an opportunity to restore my strength and mental resilience while preparing for the next round of chemotherapy. It had become increasingly challenging in the second half of my treatment plan because the cumulative effects of the chemotherapy effectively broke my body down to its weakest state. The delays set me up to recuperate and were just long enough that I could return feeling ready and better equipped to fight through the final rounds. The world around me seemed to be spiraling further and further out of control at this turbulent time, and the way I found sanity and strength was by going deeper within. Whenever I did this, I reminded myself that I was still stronger than cancer, even when my physical body said otherwise.

I think the reason the pause in treatment bothered me as much as it did was because of my intense desire to finish. I so wanted to move on and forward from this whole ordeal. Treatment setbacks felt like unwelcome interferences, further prolonging an already long and tumultuous journey.

I was growing increasingly impatient. I was physically, mentally, and spiritually depleted. One day, after yet another call from Dr. Parker informing me that we needed to postpone the next round of chemotherapy, I was feeling particularly sorry for myself.

It was a cold, dark, and rainy late April-showers morning when I received the phone call. I had just hung up the line and was staring out my bedroom window in the apartment, watching the drops of water slowly streak down the windowpane. My blue mood seemed perfectly in sync with the dreary weather.

I was grieving over how I was supposed to have been finishing cancer treatment around my 38th birthday in June. Now, after this second delay, my chemotherapy was easily going to be prolonged well into the month of July. On my calendar, I'd circled the date I'd originally expected to finish chemotherapy in red. I had survived eight rounds of chemo at this point and was already counting down to my final day, the day when my ringing the cancer bell in the infusion center would signify my hope for the future and freedom from cancer treatment.

I needed to break away from the many never-ending hospital trips. I wanted to stop repeatedly knocking my body down and out to its breaking point. I was so incredibly tired, and I wanted desperately to be done. I often daydreamed about making it to that fateful day in the summer, thinking about how, after, I would celebrate by going somewhere with my family. I fantasized about getting out into nature. I didn't want to spend another day sick in bed or at the hospital.

As I lay in bed and scrolled through photos of friends on social media, I stopped to admire one from a group of families that we used to travel with on vacations. They had just posted a photo of themselves posing in the snow outside of a cabin rental while on a group ski trip. I felt so happy for them all, but, admittedly, it also hurt. I was envious over just how lucky they all were to be able to do those kinds of things on memory-making trips. I wanted that for myself and my family again too. The kids in the picture were all laughing and smiling, some sitting on sleds and others playfully throwing snowballs. I imagined how happy my own kids would have been had we been lucky enough to do the same.

I thought about all the years before, when I had taken the freedom my good health offered for granted. Of course, I appreciated that my family had made many wonderful memories before my disease prevented us from going on trips like this, but being sick and physically incapable now was starting to wear me down in spirit. Travel was too dangerous as it interfered with my needed access to healthcare. It was also strictly against doctor's orders: the coronavirus posed danger to me and my immediate family members, especially with my being so fragile and vulnerable.

Cancer can make you feel like a prisoner in your own body. Every hindrance in treatment only added weeks to reaching that coveted light at the end of the tunnel. I had now added more than a month's extension to what had originally been scheduled as my final day of chemotherapy. The suspense around postponing when might be the end was upsetting me.

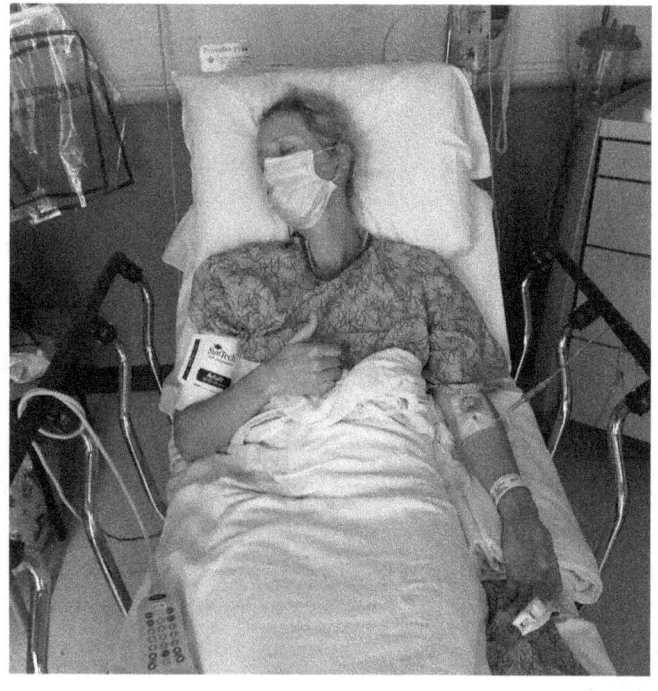

An emergency room scare.
Some days cancer treatment can get the best of you.

•••

I stared up at the rain clouds again, thinking about what I would give to go back to the warm waters of Sámara just one more time. I thought about how that trip had been the last time I had flown on an airplane. I couldn't help but wonder if that was the final flight I might ever have in my life. I thought about how, if I had known this back then, I likely would have relished the moment a little more.

I remember boarding the plane to fly home from Costa Rica, returning to Los Angeles; how, on that day, there had been a severe tropical rainstorm delaying our departure. The clouds were thick and gray, covering the horizon as far as the eye could see. Not a glimmer of sunshine was in sight. A lot like what I was now looking at in the skies above my apartment window all these months later.

I recalled how, as our plane took off that morning and made its way slowly up over the tops of the tropical green canopy of the jungle below, I had watched closely through the window, taking in the final sights of our majestic summer escape.

I felt sad as I realized our plane was entering into the cloud cover, knowing I would soon lose sight of my happy place. It officially signified the end of our summer escape. The clouds would prevent my being able to look back over a bird's eye view of paradise as we flew away from our beloved Costa Rica.

The plane's window was wet from the heavy rainstorm, and the clouds outside were thick, without any visibility. Suddenly, the plane made its way just up and out from the storm, above the clouds, into the other side of the sky. Sienna grabbed my hand while pointing out the window saying, "Mommy, look! Can you see it too? It's so beautiful."

The sun was shining brightly and illuminating the clouds now below us as we soared high above in our plane. Mother Nature was showing off one spectacular, magnificent show of sunlight. It was warm and glorious. We were perfectly timed to catch the sunrise that early morning. It felt like we had just entered heaven itself. There were white fluffy clouds streaking beneath us and colorful rays of pink, purple, and orange coming over the horizon. Of course, none of this had been visible moments before, underneath all the storm clouds now far below. This scene was only for those of us lucky enough to be on that flight, able to see what really lay just beyond the storm, and my, was this a sight to behold.

I thought about how everyone back at the airport was likely still running around in the pouring rain, trying to keep dry during the thunder and lightning. It seemed so magical that, just on the other side of that exact same cloud cover, the sun had been shining peacefully above us all along. We couldn't see it, yet it was there all along. Thinking about that final flight was the reminder I needed in that very moment so many months later.

•••

It was a reminder to me that, on what seemed like a sad morning, every storm would eventually fade and on the other side the sun would come out again to meet you. We just have to weather through until it can pass. It is said that not all storms come to disrupt your life. Some come to clear your path.

Since you can't calm the storm, my best advice is to stop trying. What you can do is calm yourself. Seek peace in the midst of the turbulence.

As I lay in bed that morning, this realization hit home. I needed to remember this lesson for myself. Even though I couldn't see or feel it from there in my bed, what I knew for certain was that indeed the sun was up there above the rain clouds, shining brightly, waiting to reappear again. Sometimes, during the greatest storms in life, you must thrust yourself forward, toward the place you are truly meant to be. I thought how maybe all of this could be true, even for me.

After the storm passes, you may not even realize how you made it through. The only thing I know for sure is that when you weather it through to reach the other side, you likely won't be the same person you were going in. And maybe that is exactly what the storm is all about. You can't enjoy the rainbow without first experiencing some rain.

I decided that I, too, was going to get through the latest setback in my treatment and weather through my next storm with unwavering hope. This delay wouldn't last forever. If I could carry through the remaining rounds to my final treatment, I, too, would have nothing but blue skies and rainbows coming my way.

> Hit a bump in the road a couple weeks back. After the results of my labs came in and needing to make several visits to the hospital - I was determined to not be strong enough to continue with chemotherapy for the time being. My oncologist decided my body needed a little break to regain some strength, recover physically and to ... See More

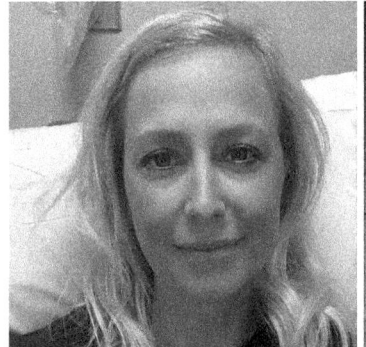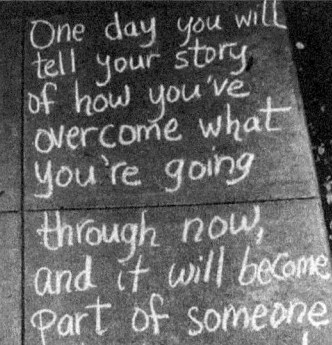

A post I shared following a pause in treatment.
One day you will tell your story of how you've overcome what you're going through now and it will become part of someone else's survival guide.

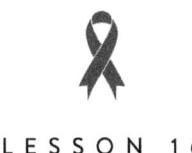

LESSON 16

YOU ARE STRONGER THAN YOU THINK

I had somehow made it through to June of 2020, concluding my eleventh round of chemotherapy. It had been eight months since that night over Thanksgiving break that I awoke with pain in my stomach. So much had happened leading up to this point, and I only had to get through the one last chemotherapy infusion of the treatment plan to finish this nightmare. I could hardly believe I had made it this far. I'd lasted for more treatments than many cancer patients on my chemotherapy regimen had been able to complete. While I did feel the impact of my grueling fight, having now grown weak and weathered, you never would have known it from the enthusiasm I was radiating. Sights set. Future-focused.

For the first time in forever things were beginning to look up. It was just before the Fourth of July holiday, and I intended to ring in the freedom this day celebrates for our great country as well as the freedom I hoped to embrace following eight harrowing months of cancer treatment. Food, fireworks, and festivities seemed more than suitable for such an occasion.

I was masterminding plans to further celebrate on that final infusion day in the weeks to come. I wanted my family and parents there when I returned home from the hospital. I was planning a delicious dinner party with cake, bright and cheery decorations, and music to dance to. We would celebrate, all together, what we all hoped would be the beginning of the end of my fight for my life against cancer.

I ordered a custom t-shirt that had a big beautiful golden bell on the front and said, "Last day of chemo!" I could hardly wait to ring that cancer bell loud and proud. At the infusion center I had celebrated with many other cancer fighters their momentous final day of treatment. It was finally going to be my turn. It was more than I could think about without happy tears of joy taking over.

I wanted nothing more than to high-five every single infusion center nurse lined up the hallway, as well as all of my fellow cancer fighters there that afternoon. I had envisioned how this moment would play out in my mind so many times. I could hardly believe this day was actually about to arrive. It was going to be epic!

Lost in so much excitement, there was a false sense of security that all was already well. It felt like we had our long overdue fresh start in life. We were unpacking from a move out of the apartment and into a house located just around the corner from my parents' home. I had just celebrated my 38th birthday, optimistic about kicking off a new year of life as a new version of me. I hoped to soon discover that all of the hard effort I had put in might have actually worked. If my prayers and wishes were answered I might possibly be lucky enough to go into remission, with no evidence of disease.

We invited my parents over for the July 4th holiday to watch fireworks in our new neighborhood. We wanted to meet some of the neighbors while safely socially distancing from our driveway. We had put our guard down, and sadly maybe a little too soon. I'm beginning to conclude that holidays in the Soto family are often muddied with unfortunate medical catastrophes. My middle son Taylor recently broke his arm in three different places from jumping off a swing set this last Easter Sunday; it required extensive surgeries, including having rods inserted, and six months of painful recovery. Thanksgiving and Christmas of this last wild year had already proven to be challenging. Now even the Fourth of July has a memory to go with it, one that will forever live up to our family's reputation for holiday misfortunes.

The day itself seemed picture-perfect, but later that night, I awoke to realize that Will was not in bed beside me. When he didn't come back from the bathroom or appear after getting a glass of water from the kitchen, I started to worry. It was two in the morning. After waiting several minutes without hearing any noise, I decided to venture downstairs and check to see where he might be. This was out of character for him, and I was concerned that something might be wrong.

I noticed a light peeking through beneath the doorway leading out into the garage and opened the door to find Will nervously pacing back-and-forth, appearing absolutely distraught. His eyes were big and bright red as though he had been crying for hours and his hair was a disheveled mess.

"Stop!" Will yelled at me once he saw me crack open the door. "Don't come any closer. You can't come in here."

I looked back at him, confused. I noticed he'd walked backward, stepping further away from me, as a response to my placing my foot onto the doorway. "What? Honey, you aren't making any sense," I said. "What's the matter?"

"Please, just stay in the house," he said. His voice was panicked. He went on to explain that he had been feeling sick for several days. We had both assumed he was having his usual bad reaction from seasonal allergies. But this night, while watching the evening news before falling asleep, he had identified an alarming new symptom, a known sign for coronavirus. A sudden loss of taste and smell was something many positive-testing COVID-19 patients were now experiencing. It was a sign you may have contracted the virus. Will had not been able to taste or smell anything for days, already, and was frightened he may now be sick and highly contagious.

Feeling beside himself that he could have contracted coronavirus, he went on to say that he would never be able to forgive himself if he had accidentally passed it on to me in my compromised state. Or the kids for that matter. All of this was clearly more than he could handle.

A test performed the next day would indeed confirm that Will was positive for COVID-19. Here's some helpful cancer advice that goes without saying: try not to catch the coronavirus!

•••

It was only a matter of hours until my symptoms began. The virus quickly attacked my system and did so with a vengeance. It was no secret that those with underlying medical conditions, including cancer, were at an increased risk.

This happened early enough during the pandemic that there still was much unknown by the medical community for how best to treat hospitalized patients. It was during that first summer surge here in the United States. Even less was known around how to treat cancer patients who contracted the virus at that time. Doctors warned about those with pre-existing conditions being critically susceptible to the virus, and cancer patients were obviously some of the most defenseless of all.

Cancer treatment that suppresses the immune system—such as chemotherapy—leaves patients risking extreme reactions to coronavirus without the ability to defend themselves. Cancer patients have a higher likelihood of severe illness from COVID-19 by having a weakened immune system.

After eight months of treatment and eleven rounds of chemotherapy my immune system was practically nonexistent. My latest labs had shown my having a dangerously low white blood cell count, below the charts, as in zero. My body's ability to fight infection had been weakened by immunosuppression, and the doctors said I was neutropenic.

Neutropenia is defined as a lower-than-normal number of neutrophils (a type of white blood cell). White blood cells are part of the immune system. There are different types of white blood cells, and they each play a key role in the body's defense against germs. They form a very important defense against most types of infection.

Normally, most of our white blood cells are neutrophils. In patients with cancer, neutropenia is usually caused by treatment. When looking at your risk of getting an infection, doctors look at the number of neutrophils you have. For people with cancer, having a low neutrophil count is the biggest risk factor for getting a serious infection. Contracting the virus or any infection in my weakened condition was considered extremely dangerous and couldn't have happened at a worse time.

My symptoms started with a sore throat, earache, fever, and headache. Within hours I had grown so weak I could hardly open my eyes and was even losing consciousness. By the time I was admitted to the hospital, I was already incredibly sick, so much so that I required assistance from a security guard to lift my frail body out from the passenger seat of my mom's car. He gently placed me into a wheelchair and they rushed me to the COVID-19 tent located just outside of the emergency room.

My mom explained to the security guard helping push my wheelchair and the nurse who was admitting me that my husband had just tested positive for COVID-19, that I was now exhibiting symptoms, and that I was an advanced Stage 3 cancer patient. The nurse exclaimed, "Oh shit!" I'm sure she hadn't meant to actually say it aloud. It was a shocked response.

I was too weak to open my eyes or speak up for myself, but hearing the nurse respond in horror over my fragile state and dangerous prognosis was only the tip of the iceberg for what was soon to come. Within an hour my test results came back positive for COVID-19. I was whisked away to the ICU COVID wing in the most debilitating state of health I'd reached in all of my life.

I believe I was the first cancer patient treated for coronavirus in the ICU at the hospital. The doctor said they were still learning how to treat patients with coronavirus, and he, at least, had not yet treated a cancer patient. I was his first. We all knew I was severely at risk. I would come closer to death from COVID-19 than I had at any point as an advanced colorectal cancer patient receiving chemotherapy. The virus viciously attacked my immunocompromised body, leaving me with little to no defense, no ability to fight back. It was not a very promising position to be in.

During my time in the ICU, I reached my lowest of lows. Looking back, I now see this as the pivotal turning point in my entire story. It was the time where I had to put everything I'd been practicing and preaching, everything I'd been preparing for, to this final test. I'd finished my cancer treatment because I was now battling coronavirus. It was one hell of a grand finale.

•••

My life literally was hanging on the line and depended on my getting all I had learned over the course of cancer down right. The strong medications pumping through my IV line were not powerful enough for my frail body to respond to. I was quickly going from bad to worse and starting to fail to thrive. I don't actually recall much of the first three days in ICU, as I was in and out of consciousness, awakening only when a nurse came in to check my vitals.

They had explained to me that COVID-19 patients in intensive care were considered such a high risk to encounter that we were isolated. We were very much alone. Nurses and doctors came into your room only when absolutely necessary, donning full personal protective equipment (PPE). This was far more than my infusion center nurses' usual protective gear. Coronavirus ICU health care professionals had to wear protective clothing and astronaut-like head masks with breathing tubes. They looked like they were suiting up for an extraterrestrial battle, preparing to approach an alien on another planet. I, of course, was the alien.

Every time anyone entered my room, they would gown up and glove up and then carefully disinfect their gown and gloves; they threw it all away upon exiting. Nothing could be repurposed due to my dangerous germs.

PPE materials were so low in supply due to COVID's summer surge that they had to avoid coming into your room unless it was absolutely vital. I wasn't given the usual hospital bedside remote with a red call button; rather, I was told to use the telephone so that nobody would have to enter the room to turn off the remote's call alarm. My IV line was long and ran from my hand to outside my closed, isolated room. My medications and other equipment were safely stored outside, too, for nurses to access from the hallway. It reminded me a lot of that movie *Outbreak*. I was the super infectious, sick patient trapped inside a bubble, safely isolated from the world while fighting for my life.

I slept through the first few days and honestly barely recall very much at all other than briefly waking up, confused, to discover 12 hours had passed in what felt like the blink of an eye. Each time I awoke, I felt weaker and found myself gasping to breathe air. My nurses were so incredibly caring, and they no doubt worked tirelessly to care for more patients than the hospital could handle. Many of my nurses weren't typically ICU nurses, but they filled in as the unit was over capacity. The COVID ICU wing was so full that they were opening another one to meet the high demand for care of too many patients with life-threatening needs. The nurses couldn't spend much time with me, but when they did enter my room, I would catch some praying over me. Others generously stayed awhile, risking their safety to visit with me a little longer in an effort to comfort me. They were all so heroic.

I would wake up some nights to hear other ICU patients crying out in agony from the rooms down the hall; they couldn't breathe. I heard "Code Blue 5th Floor ICU" called out over the PA system repeatedly, indicating the critical status of my neighboring patients in the unit. As the days passed, fluid continued to fill my lungs and breathing became increasingly harder. The doctors were trying the few potent drugs available that could support me as my diminished immune system fought the virus, but my frail body was not responding.

I had to dig deeper than ever before and find invisible strength within to discover power even I didn't realize I had. For several days I continued to decline and was starting to fail to thrive.

One morning the nurse had me turn to lie on my stomach. I was struggling to breathe because of the fluid now pooling in my lungs; they hoped changing my position could help. I overheard my doctor and nurse speaking outside of my room that day. If I didn't start to respond within the next 24 hours, they would consider putting me onto supplemental oxygen.

I had watched enough of the news to know that this was a bad sign. I realized that, if this did happen, it meant I would likely grow weaker and sicker—not to mention that my risk for developing an infection was increasing. My body did not have the strength to handle the challenges confronting it. This was life-threatening. The number of ICU patients dying each day from the virus was terrifying and knowing I soon could join the growing statistic only added to my fear. At this time, in the summer of 2020, most COVID-19 ICU patients stayed for an average of six weeks or more, fighting for their lives, with many on breathing machines. Many did not survive. My survival was on the line, and I knew it.

The game plan was to let me sleep through one more night and make a decision come the morning. They would review my next chest x-ray and determine whether my oxygen levels and other lab results were or weren't starting to show signs of improvement.

• • •

When I woke up the next morning, I struggled to breathe now more than ever before, and the panic started settling in quickly. I wasn't getting better.

"This is it. You're done now," I thought to myself. "I was already at a disadvantage when I first caught this. I came here too broken and weak from cancer to beat this. The doctor's reports sound hopeless. I am starting to fail quickly, moving in the wrong direction with every passing day. I am barely able to breathe, and the reason I am now gasping for air is that I am about to be taken down and out, once and for all. This is really it. This is how I am going to die. Might as well stop fighting it. Certainly, nobody will blame me. I am just so tired. I put up a valiant effort but have grown weary. Maybe it is time to finally allow myself to rest. I should give in. Time to surrender. Let it happen. Stop fighting back and go in peace."

The last eight months of being in a constant state of fight or flight had taken their toll. Not seeing my beloved family since being admitted into Intensive Care was shattering my soul. Cancer had already beaten me down, and now the virus was too intense. It had become unbearable. I couldn't fight for breath another day. I was sick. I was tired. I was alone. I am not ashamed to admit it: that was the one day I lost my will to live.

Thoughts of doubt now plagued my mind. I had told my family, all the months before this, that I was going to do absolutely everything in my power to survive. But without my ability to see them, to hug them, to have them there with me now when I needed them the most, I was struggling. They were not there to remind me of all the powerful thoughts and words I had spoken, my belief in victory over defeat. And now even I was losing all hope.

I wondered if maybe I was supposed to have died from cancer and had somehow cheated fate. Possibly, and if so, had I somehow managed to buy myself a little more time, but now destiny was catching up? Maybe this was why I was now so sick from the coronavirus? Because cancer hadn't killed me when it was supposed to, would COVID-19 be what finally sealed the deal for my destiny with death?

I honestly don't think I'd be here today if I hadn't decided to use what minuscule amount of reserve I had left that morning to make what I believed might be my final phone call to my family. I did so out of the fear that, if I needed to go onto breathing assistance later that day, I wouldn't be well enough to speak to them ever again.

Maybe I'd grown so sick I wouldn't be able to call them on my cell phone this time tomorrow. I already could barely hold the phone long enough to dial home. It dawned on me that I may never hear or see my family again. Never have the pleasure of their warm embrace. No chance to kiss the tops of my babies' sweet heads of hair. I wished I had held onto them all a little longer before leaving for the emergency room. It all had happened so quickly. I didn't realize at the time, but that moment may have been our final goodbye. This phone call was my way of telling them how much I loved them - in case it was the last chance I ever could.

Typing this out doesn't adequately tell what this moment was like in actual reality. That phone call was the hardest thing I've ever had to do, harder than all the cancer and tougher than fighting COVID-19. The emotions it carried were incredibly intense. I called using Facetime so I that could not only hear but see them. My hands were weak. My pillow was propped up against the hospital bed and I laid my phone against it so that I could at least watch them on the screen. I was careful to intentionally position the screen to show only below my neckline. I didn't want them seeing my face. I was afraid they would see me as a failure, and I did not want that image to be their final memory of who I am.

I could barely speak from all the fluid inside of my chest and was gasping for every breath. I cried into the pillow, but even crying hurt my lungs so much that it too was hard to manage. I listened to them intensely after they answered my call, gathered together and seated on our family sofa, telling me about our cat, Shadow, and how they had had waffles for breakfast. Each of the kids was talking a million miles a minute, trying to catch me up on everything I had missed back at home while away in the hospital.

I could barely see the phone screen, which upset me because I didn't want to miss looking at their beautiful faces, but I was too weak to raise my hand to even wipe the tears from my eyes and refocus. It lifted every ounce of my soul to just hear the sweet sound of their voices on the other end of that line. All I wanted at that moment was to listen to those I love most in the entire world.

Will must have heard me crying from the other side. Either that, or he had noticed how I wasn't able to speak or answer their many questions. Somehow, he figured out that something was terribly wrong. He grabbed the phone from the kids and rushed into the bedroom, safely away from them, insisting that I hold up the phone to show him my face.

"I can't," I tried to say while choking on my words.

"Yes, you can," he said. "Please. Don't you dare do this, Erin. Why are you, of all people, giving up?" he said. "Not you. Not today. This is not how our story ends. You haven't come this far to only make it this far. Where is my wife? I need you to come back to me, please." Will was now crying along with me on the other end of the line. After seeing my face, he instantly knew in his heart that I had finally given up my fight to live.

"I need you to get up. Don't you give up on us. Not yet. You are so much stronger than even you realize."

He proceeded to give me what I consider possibly the greatest pep talk in all the universe. He reminded me how I was the one always talking about the power of mindset being our greatest medicine. I talked all this talk, now walk the walk. Time to practice what I preached. Time to put myself to the greatest test of all. A test I had been preparing for all this time, and that I could manage with the grace of God. He then spoke unconditional love, unwavering strength, power, greatness, and healing into me.

He pleaded with me again to not give up on the life we had built together. He reminded me of my many whys, all the reasons I truly wanted to live for and had yet to experience. He begged me to at least try one last time to do this for him and our four beloved babies who still need their mommy. He then told me I needed to stand up. Rise out of that hospital bed. He ordered me to move, to walk, and then use the day to regain my stamina and strength.

I needed this moment with Will. This was the day we decided together that I was going to recover and make it back home to my family. No matter what.

Will didn't care that I didn't feel like it, or that I believed I lacked the physical, emotional, and spiritual strength to do so. He told me he knew I could do this because I had promised him I would, all that time before. I had already done too many extraordinary things and had overcome so many odds. I surely would have one powerful story to tell to serve as an example to others that they, too, are capable of exactly the same. And now, he needed me to fulfill all the bold promises I had made to my entire family. He instructed me to show up and rise above what I felt and all the excuses. It was time to prove to everyone what I was made of. Even if I was doing so isolated in that damn ICU room, all alone, he knew I was capable of so much more in life. He only needed me to see the incredible strength within that I had somehow lost sight of for myself.

There is no question that the phone call saved my life. I committed then and there to see myself differently than the way I felt. I refused to accept the doubt and concern my doctors had about my prognosis. I refused to listen to my now failing weak and sickly body. I decided to place all my faith over all my fear and believe in myself again, even with all the odds stacked against me.

There's so much power in mindset, prayer, belief, hope, and possibility. As long as you choose to acknowledge and recognize it. I know this is true. I wasn't allowed to give up. Not this way. It took everything I had left, but that morning I stood up for the first time in days and got out of the hospital bed. I set off the bed alarm when doing so, much to the horror of my ICU nurse, who came rushing in after taking a minute to throw on her PPE gear faster than I'd seen yet. I was an extreme fall risk after so many days spent in the hospital bed. She took one look at my tear-stained face and saw my fight for life and my determination. She stopped talking mid-sentence to let me say what I was insistent on her understanding. It was clear to her that I wasn't going to listen to what she said about my needing to get safely back to bed. I told her I was going to be going home later that week, and first we needed to stand me up and start to move in order for me to regain my strength.

Over the course of the next day, I somehow managed to slowly stand, then sit outside of my bed, and then walk. Within 24 hours I somehow started to respond to treatment, and I know this is only because my will to live and decision to do so allowed my body to fall into alignment with my head and my heart.

The doctors tell me what happened in that room, with my being a sick cancer patient who seemingly managed to turn around suddenly, finally responding to all of the powerful treatment overnight, was like nothing they had seen yet. It took several days more, but I continued to slowly improve. After only one week in the ICU, a cancer patient, no less, when nobody else was faring the same, I was given the approval for discharge and told I could return home to recover. It was too risky to keep me there in my condition, but also incredibly far from what they saw as cleared. I had a long road of recovery yet to make, but I was getting better. The doctors told me that what happened to me in that hospital room was nothing short of a miracle.

It turned out that the drugs they used to treat me soon became the standard treatment used to help COVID-19 patients turn around more quickly than had been seen up to this point. But that still doesn't explain how it managed to work as quickly as it did with my unique cancer-riddled body and extreme circumstances.

It had taken another four very long emotionally and physically grueling days of hard work and determination before I was eventually given the grace of enough restored health to return to my family and my home. The discharge nurse arrived at my room, helped me into my wheelchair, and took me out to the hallway. It was a scene just like out of a movie.

The nurse tapped my shoulder gently and whispered into my ear, "Erin, look up. This is all for you!" I could hear music start to play on the speakers in the hallway and saw that every single ICU nurse was standing there smiling back at me with thumbs up and high fives as I was wheeled by, singing along to Journey's *Don't Stop Believin'* that was now blaring on the speaker system.

I realized the date was the same day I was supposed to have finished my final chemotherapy infusion. This day and its victory were even more epic than my vision of ringing the cancer bell back at the infusion center. This was indeed my grand finale. I knew it. I had not only just crushed cancer but Coronavirus too, much to the delight of myself and the many heroes working tirelessly in the hospital to save the lives of so many. In the movie *Wonder,* Auggie Pullman famously said that "Everyone in the world should get a standing ovation at least once in their life." Well, my standing ovation was one for the history books. It was even more glorious than I had dreamed for.

We all cried and sang together in unison as my nurse slowly wheeled me out. The head ICU nurse chased me down to tell me that, from the time I had been admitted, she had been praying for my family and me. As a mother herself, she had seen so much suffering and too much loss. She said that watching me not only survive against such odds but recover as quickly as I had somehow managed to do, brought the glimmer of hope the staff all so needed to keep going on as they fought against this dreadful virus.

What I did that week in the ICU was nothing short of monumental. I share it to remind you of how powerful you are, too. You were born with everything you need to defeat whatever is trying to stop you. You, too, were created to overcome. You came into this life perfectly designed and well equipped to take on the most daunting crises and circumstances life throws your direction. Even the ones you never believed you would have the courage or strength to survive.

You may feel weak, fragile, and intimidated even, but don't ever let the way you feel blind you from your innate personal power. You, too, are a magnificent warrior. Don't let your feelings of doubt have the final say. You have to go by only what you know.

I could've listened to that voice in my head. I could have given up. At the time, that certainly seemed like the easy thing to do. I knew I was at a great disadvantage as a cancer patient. I knew I looked small, felt insignificant, and was also very sick. But I'm a fighter. I'm a mother. I'm a wife. I'm so much stronger than I look.

I've got more inside of me than meets the eye. I've got something extraordinary deep within. My love for my family gave me the will to live and the power I needed to fight back one more time.

It's easy to get discouraged when facing things you don't understand. To give up on your dreams, to ask why this is happening to you. But that is what's going to keep you from persevering. That's not the right attitude and not the right mindset.

The situation you are facing may seem unbearable. The overwhelm and pain may appear too daunting to overcome.

The thing is, this problem you are facing wasn't placed here to stop you from arriving at your destination. It's often what is going to carry you to it.

Cancer and COVID-19 weren't brought here to defeat me but were there to help me discover the power that has lain within. The best part, I believe, is that each and every time you outlast and endure another life crisis you are setting yourself up for new levels of promotion. You aren't going to come out the other side of this the same person you were going into it. You are going to grow through it all.

The most important takeaway from my grand COVID-19 finale is that, without everything that happened to me, I would never have had the opportunity to reach my fullest potential.

There are going to be times in life where you don't feel courageous and determined, but simply overwhelmed, and you may lose hope and start to give in to defeat. Especially in your fight with cancer. When that happens, though, you need to be stronger than your strongest excuse.

Deep down inside, I had somehow known this day was coming. It's what I'd been preparing for all along my journey until this fateful moment arrived. I knew that this was my time to become everything I was created to be. I knew that I was not only just going to survive cancer but going to conquer coronavirus, too. I knew I was going to get out of the hospital. I knew I was going to regain my strength and recover my health.

I knew that the purpose for all of this would be for me to one day share my story and use it to prove to others that they, too, are equally capable of overcoming whatever adversity they are facing in their own life.

And now it's your turn. You, too, are a history maker. You, too, are a glorious fighter. You are capable of far more than you realize. You are not just going to survive; you are going to thrive. You, too, are going to overcome every obstacle and defeat set before you. I am stronger than cancer, and you are stronger than you know. You only need to believe in yourself as much as I do.

Irvine Medical Center.
Jul 12, 2020 · Irvine

I am going to share a happy ending to what has been a nightmare of a week. That is an understatement. Those who know me understand I've already been through one hell of an 8 month battle starting with my cancer diagnosis, surgeries, chemo and kicking cancers butt - ...TO NOW ALSO HAVING SURVIVED COVID!! 😳

I never knew how strong 💪 I actually was, b... See More

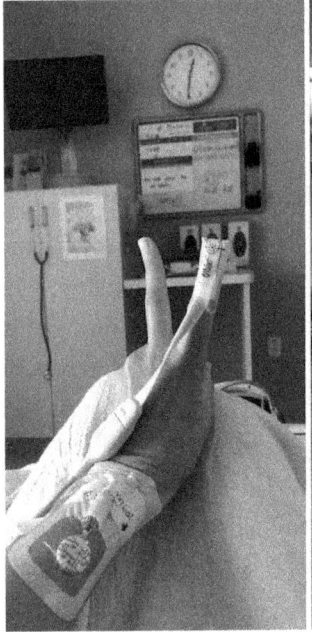
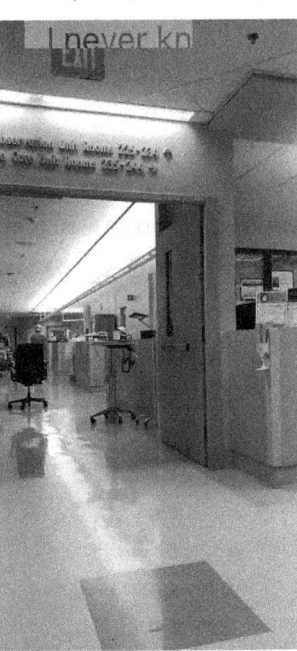

A post shared the day I was discharged from the intensive care unit (ICU) for COVID-19.

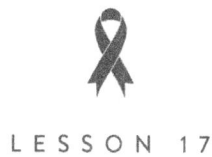

LESSON 17

BELIEVE IN YOUR ABILITY TO THRIVE

Returning home from the hospital was just as elated a reunion as I'm sure you can imagine. To be able to see my husband and my children after everything I had just been through in the intensive care unit was truly one of the greatest highlights in all of my life.

The caveat was that we were to quarantine in our house together for the next 14 days as we were, understandably, deemed contagious and at risk of passing the coronavirus to others.

As the days passed, I slowly continued to regain strength. Not surprisingly, my oncologist advised I miss the final twelfth round of chemotherapy that I had been scheduled to attend since I was clearly not in any shape or condition to withstand further cancer treatment. The damage the coronavirus had done to my body and immune system, paired with the cumulative impact of cancer treatment, made it far too dangerous to complete that last chemotherapy infusion.

Dr. Parker endearingly told me that I have not been anything like a typical cancer patient, and that my latest surprise in battling Coronavirus after 11 rounds of chemotherapy was certainly one for the record books! To go through this in my condition had given him, and all of my doctors, quite the scare. He also knew I was one hell of a fighter and was honored to celebrate the official end of my cancer treatment and how I managed to make it as far as I did. It was some journey, and apparently, now was the long-awaited time for me to finally rest.

"Just like that?" I thought to myself. "After everything that I've been through? The nonstop fighting for my life over the course of the last eight months, is it really all over? I'm actually done?"

"What am I supposed to do now?" I asked Dr. Parker.

He explained that we were going into what he calls 'surveillance mode.' This is the time after treatment where the body gets to take a much-needed break from constant doctors' visits, battering from ongoing treatment, and all else we cancer patients are put through. I'd endured more than enough.

I should now slowly recover over the course of the next several months. He added I might even start to feel almost back to my old self as time goes on. Of course, he explained, we wouldn't know if any of the treatment we had done was successful until I passed my post-treatment colonoscopy and cancer scan, and this couldn't happen for several months' time.

It required going into a waiting game to watch and see what happens. Until then, he advised I try to go back to my 'normal' life and appreciate the freedom that having wrapped treatment offered. I had finished, officially, and our hope is it will remain that way. He added that my hard work in fighting cancer just might, indeed, have finally come to an end. I had crossed the finish line! Celebrating this momentous achievement was in order, despite it being something only time could tell.

I was ecstatic! My family and I threw one wild celebration, a festive party where together we laughed, we cried, we ate, we danced, and we sang in jubilation. This cancer ordeal might actually be over. Or then again, was it?

I was thrilled to have made it this far in the journey, yet I now had to somehow manage to wait months in order to find out if the hell storm I'd battled my way through had even worked. The jubilation I experienced was short-lived and, not long after, I found myself feeling lost and confused all over again.

We had celebrated my outlasting and surviving cancer treatment and coronavirus, being formally cleared as having no evidence of disease

(NED). But am I really a 'cancer survivor'? Technically speaking, according to many, I am only 'in remission.' My highest risk of recurrence is now, in this first year. Then my risk slowly reduces with each year I pass as cancer-free, and I will only be deemed a "survivor" after making it through a five-year term.

That doesn't mean cancer can't recur beyond five years. Certain cancers can recur many years after first being treated. For some cancers, if it has not returned by five years after initial diagnosis, the chance of a later recurrence is very small; but the way I see it, every one of us is at risk every darn day.

As far as I'm concerned, I am a cancer survivor and was from the very moment that I was diagnosed. As is the way I view everyone else with this disease, for that matter. You are a survivor as long as you have been diagnosed with cancer and are still living. If that is you, then you are "one of us." Welcome to the survivor's club!

Despite having wrapped treatment and feeling like I was a true survivor moving on in life, going back to usual activities was not possible after having gone through such extensive treatment following a traumatic crisis. I was told to resume my normal ways in life. Easier said than done. I had to ask myself what normal even meant anymore. I wasn't sure.

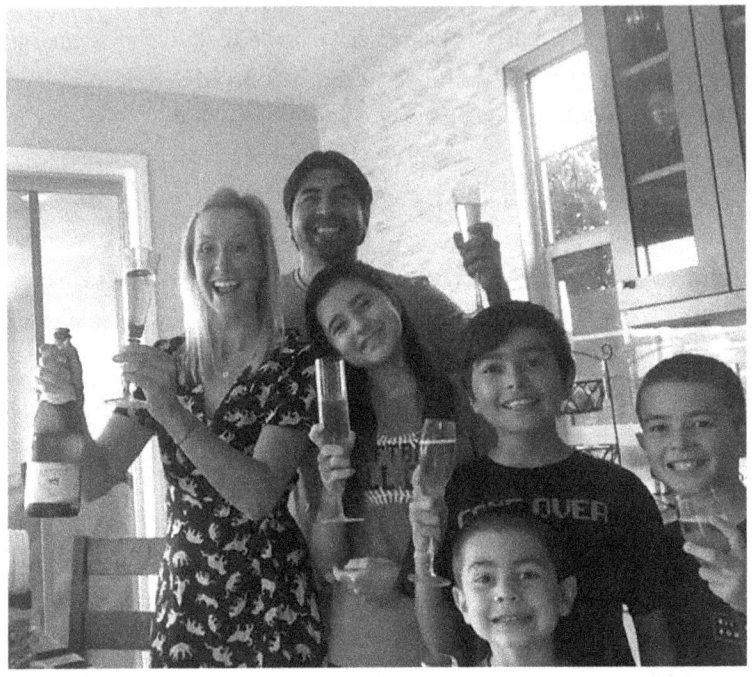

Pop, fizz, clink! We celebrated the end of cancer treatment and Coronavirus by sipping champagne and sparkling cider.

What Is Normal?

I certainly couldn't go back to life as it was before cancer. That somehow had gotten me here in the first place. Besides, I had changed substantially and was not the same person I was the day cancer crashed into my life.

Facing forward and moving on with life after cancer can feel like sunshine mixed with a little hurricane. Although you are glad it's over, you also wonder about what may come next. You feel you shouldn't quite let your guard down and celebrate too much, too soon, or the ball may drop, and a cancer recurrence will come to crash your party.

The fear that cancer might come back and a newfound appreciation for the fragility of life, paired with a new perspective on death and dying, well, that all together is all a heavy burden to live with.

Most people are likely to adapt well after treatment ends and they resume usual routines; but that happens over time. For many, it is common to experience ongoing fears and concerns. You may find you need a lot of support—possibly even more support than you did when you were first diagnosed or during treatment.

Emotions that were brushed aside during treatment may come flooding back all at once, and you might find yourself feeling overwhelmed with fear, sadness, and anger all over again, just as you did with the post-diagnosis grieving process. You experience delayed reactions that come out of nowhere.

Many people do not expect negative emotions once their treatment ends, and I certainly found this all to be really confusing. Along with the fear and sadness, I was in an overall heightened emotional state. I might get tearful and reactive very quickly, particularly after being asked how I was feeling. I might say, "I'm okay, I think. I don't know, actually. Now I'm crying! Why does this keep happening?"

There were days a couple of months after where I might experience frustration because I felt as though my family and friends expected too much from me. I wasn't ready to tackle certain responsibilities but felt pressured to take on more than I knew I ought to. Because I appeared healthy, many assumed I was right as rain and perfectly equipped to get back into action at the level I had before treatment. I found I was not physically or emotionally able to do some of the things I had before cancer.

I also had (still have) survivor guilt creep up on me at times. I find myself feeling guilty or questioning why I survived cancer when others didn't. This can feel pretty confounding to face whenever it happens.

Above all, I mostly felt as if my body and spirit were now tired and what I needed was a lot of rest and plenty of time to recover. It had been such a long time since I could just relax. It felt foreign and weird to adjust to. I inherently knew I shouldn't push myself or jump back in too quickly or too soon.

All of these feelings make perfect sense. Cancer survivors wrapping treatment have just been through a tumultuous season. You've had to make major life decisions. Your body has been assaulted by cancer and its treatment. Your perspective on life has drastically changed.

Just as it was following diagnosis, facing these feelings and learning how to deal with them all over again when they bubble up to the surface is important. Don't expect everything to go back to the way it was before you were diagnosed. Just like it took time to adjust to life with cancer, you will adjust to life after cancer, but that won't likely happen overnight.

This applies to your family, too. Give yourself, your family, and everyone around you time. You'll get through this. You may find that your former pre-cancer identity and role in your home and family life may continue to change. You might want to embrace adjustments that occurred during treatment. I'm talking about those many things that you did before having cancer that, since, were being done by others.

Maybe some tasks you'll want to take back. Possibly, in areas where others have stepped up to new roles, they won't be willing to give your former responsibility back to you. And for the items that are put back onto your plate, they maybe aren't given the same priority or sense of urgency they once held before.

Let me tell you, today I am busier than ever as a wife, mom of four, and daughter, caring for the family members who live in my home while also helping my parents who live up the street. But my bar and expectations now are far lower than they used to be before cancer. I refuse to sweat the small stuff.

I am also happy to report that my four kids also seem to have bounced back, as in laughing more often and appearing relaxed, comfortable, and far less anxious. It's taken them time to get here, though, and we all know too well that life can throw an unexpected curveball at any given moment. We are all so appreciative for each and every good day we are blessed with. Now more than ever before.

The last thing I personally struggled with was feeling that many of the people, social circles, and settings I used to enjoy no longer appealed to me after cancer. I have found that people who tend to keep conversations superficial, have a habit of complaining about small stuff problems, or lack awareness, compassion, depth, or genuine authenticity quickly bore me. I still enjoy small talk, of course, but the people to whom I feel drawn today are often ones who share in holding an intentional life perspective and connection with others. I was a lot less harsh of a critic before cancer than I find myself being now. I don't mean this in a negative way; it's just that I am protective over who and where I give my time and energy to.

The core circle I surround myself with continues to grow and change as I evolve into life after cancer. I find this to be one of the most noticeable changes after re-entering the real world. I've got big dreams to chase, goals to achieve, and many hopes to fulfill in order to leave a lasting legacy that I can "rest in peace" with in case I encounter an early expiration date in life.

I truly try to live each day without regrets going on into the next. That coveted second chance I desperately prayed for and got: I refuse to waste it and I intend to fulfill the promises I made. Of course, every day can't revolve around changing the world in big ways, and I relish the many little miracles too.

I guess I understood after wrapping treatment that I was embarking on a new chapter in life after cancer, one that can bring hope and happiness but is strangely tainted with plenty of new worries and fears I never carried before.

Going back to "normal" is a period of adjustment that takes a lot of time. Living with the anxiety, after treatment, of not knowing if it was successful; wondering about the risk for recurrence; and trying to casually make your way back into life is so much easier said than done.

Let's highlight some of the most common feelings cancer survivors I know seem to experience. This is meant to better prepare for the road ahead around what to expect should you be someone recently finishing cancer treatment or living as a fellow survivor in remission. I think it is important to note the difficulties I faced in navigating life after cancer, as much of this was rather unexpected.

Scanxiety

The fear of cancer coming back (called cancer recurrence) is common among cancer survivors and can sometimes be quite intense. Many cancer survivors feel anxious before follow-up appointments, as going in to check for cancer understandably causes a lot of emotions and memories to boil to the surface, bringing them up to process all over again.

This is such a common feeling there is even a term for it. "Scanxiety" is a word used in the cancer world to describe the tension which builds as you move towards your post-treatment or annual cancer scan. "Hyper-scanxiety" only exacerbates this further and follows having just completed your cancer scan; it describes how you feel during the time that elapses as you await results.

To boot, there is another common experience that comes after you receive your results. I'm not sure what to label this one, but it's definitely a widespread emotion that many can relate to. I call it the "Cancer Coaster Ride." For reference, let me share what this feels like.

I had my first post-cancer treatment colonoscopy in late November of 2020, precisely one year following that fateful Thanksgiving of 2019 diagnosis.

I was a nervous wreck and so worked up this time around that the twilight anesthesia didn't work as it had before. I was wide awake and alert for the entire colonoscopy. I told my doctor that I wanted to hear and see whatever they did in real time. I was thankful when the gastroenterologist held my hand and told me I had just passed with no evidence of cancer. What a relief! I could not avoid tearing up, considering how tragically this same test had gone for me that last time. I was in the same exam room, the same health center, and, of course, couldn't avoid reliving that horrible diagnosis memory from one year before. The relief I felt after passing was monumental, but I was far from done.

I still had to pass the cancer scan, where they checked to see if the cancer had crept up anywhere else in my body, spreading outside of my colon. Remember those two lymph nodes that tested positive, resulting in my needing chemotherapy? This was to test for that!

I was so, so anxious before that first scan. I made the terrible mistake of attending my daughter's softball tournament the weekend before, thinking the escape of watching her team compete in games outside in the fresh air would somehow help keep my mind off the insanity I was experiencing in my heart. I practically bit off two softball parent friends' heads when they tried to take Sienna's sandwich order in between games.

In hindsight, I was a hot mess who never should have left my house that weekend. I know that everyone there on the field with us that day likely thought I was another crazy softball mom but, in reality, I was a shaken cancer patient falling fully apart in plain sight in dreaded anticipation for that coming Tuesday's cancer scan.

I found myself hoping and praying the scan would be clear, all while wondering how I would cope if it was not. How would I tell people if something was indeed wrong? Could I survive going back for ongoing treatment if I had to?

It's the scariest roller coaster ride that only cancer patients know about. This Cancer Coaster isn't the kind of thrill you want to experience first-hand. I was trying to hope for the best while preparing for the worst.

After I completed my scary scan and learned the results (all clear and no evidence of disease!), I fell into another whirlwind of bizarre emotions. I had to reach out to fellow cancer survivors for moral support to help with coping. Trust me, although they try, non-cancer friends just can't understand what it is like when it comes to re-entering life after cancer. The struggle is real.

If you are fortunate enough to pass the cancer test, it's only a brief reprieve. You come to recognize that this relief, this false sense of security and safety, is only temporarily lived. You'll do it all over again in six months, one year, two years, or whatever your doctor has ordered. For many, this will continue for the rest of your life. It's never really ever over, but if you are healthy enough to keep passing your scans and extending the time between the next, it does eventually get a little easier with time.

Post-Traumatic Stress

I have even experienced symptoms of post-traumatic stress. For cancer survivors, this usually begins within the first three months after the trauma but can also not appear until months or even years afterward. In other words, cancer survivors and their families will need long-term monitoring.

Post-traumatic stress disorder (PTSD) is an anxiety disorder. A person may develop PTSD after experiencing a frightening or life-threatening situation. PTSD is often associated with war, physical attacks, natural disasters, and serious accidents. People with cancer experience it too.

A study by researchers at the Herbert Irving Comprehensive Cancer Center at Columbia University Medical Center found that nearly 1 in 4 women newly diagnosed with breast cancer experienced PTSD.

Memories from my cancer experience that seem to trigger PTSD include having ongoing cancer tests and visiting the hospital site where I received cancer treatment. On one recent visit, I sat in the parking lot of the hospital while salivating and spitting onto the ground, trying not to vomit for at least fifteen minutes. I was experiencing that nausea I'd felt with my former chemotherapy, but this was more than six months after treatment. I was there to take my son for a regular pediatric check-up, yet I found myself having a strange after-attack from cancer treatment; it was caused by mental association and memory with the location. We waited a good twenty minutes before I could pull myself together enough to walk inside the building.

I don't think I've ever visited the hospital again without staring up at my window on the fifth floor, recalling my time spent in the Intensive Care Unit. I can see the very window I looked out of on the summer day, suffering with Coronavirus, when I decided to fight back for my life. I relive the memory of the kind nurse who, after that call to my family, let me lean on her arm for support, intent on completing the ten small steps it took to look out of that very window. That window symbolizes one of the scariest and most victorious days in my life.

Last week, I met with my oncologist on the fourth floor of the same hospital to check in and order my upcoming one-year cancer scans. I found myself wandering down the hallway from the clinic waiting area toward the infusion center and, for no good reason, sitting in the exact chair of the infusion center waiting area that I sat in on my first day of chemotherapy. I was overwhelmed with emotion and started to cry as I recalled my hands shaking while sitting there not so long ago, terrified of what was to come. I didn't at first notice that a young woman had taken a seat just behind me. She had on a purple headscarf and was clearly there waiting for cancer treatment. She tried to give me her best, encouraging smile, likely assuming I was afraid.

Just at that moment, one of my favorite infusion center nurses happened to walk by and recognized me, stopping in shock to find me sitting, out of place, at the infusion center waiting area. She was the nurse who had told me on my first day of chemotherapy that I was one of the ones she expected to make it, based on my strong will to live. She asked how I was doing and joked about how happy she was not to have seen me around these parts for such a long time.

"My last chemotherapy was just over a year ago," I said. "Don't worry. I'm not here for treatment today. I somehow wandered down this side of the hall while lost in thought, I guess." We then hugged and celebrated my remission status together, since I never got the chance to ring the cancer bell.

My name was then called, and I needed to walk back down the hallway to the other waiting room, the one where patients sit to meet with their oncologists. I stood up and peered through the open door of the infusion center as my former favorite nurse entered inside. I turned around and started to walk away, giving a reassuring smile back to the lady sitting behind me. I whispered to her as I walked: "If I could do this, I know you can too."

...

Dr. Parker kindly asked if I wanted to wait until January to avoid putting myself and my family through the whirlwind of cancer scans during the holiday season. We'd had no choice but to go through that for the last two years. He let me know that if I preferred, considering my condition, I could wait a few extra weeks and push my scans to January. In hindsight, I'm questioning if I should have taken him up on the offer to delay that next cancer scan, but I told him I have a book to publish and life to live come January. This Thanksgiving I will be back at it, hoping to have passed one more scan that buys me another year of freedom. While I have no guarantee that all will go well, I'm cautiously optimistic.

I've made it this far for a reason. I've also done so much, over the last eight months, in writing this book. This next year ahead holds work I have yet to complete for my advocacy work for colon cancer patients. Ideally, I will continue working on as a cancer survivor, not as an active patient.

As I type this page, it is early October 2021. I admit there has been a sense of urgency behind finishing this final chapter so I can publish this book and do so quickly. I shared with you before that I started writing the week after passing my cancer scan around Christmas 2020, and I've been pouring my heart out onto these pages ever since.

I can only pray this book serves its intended purpose of helping the many it was written to serve. I also hope to be here, alive and well, my health intact and ideally cancer-free, to experience and relish in the pivotal day it's published. I also respect the possibility that looms in my coming cancer tests and the uncertainty for my future.

I am working tirelessly to finish this book on time, in case the worst-case scenario happens, but I'm wishing only for the best. If you are reading this today, it means I published this book! And regardless of what happens to me around my health, please send a prayer and note of encouragement. If you've followed my recounting my journey this far, you deserve a personal thank you from me. I gladly welcome reaching out on social media or over an email where we can share well wishes and thoughts with one another.

In the coming months, I hope to celebrate my one-year survivorship. It is a huge milestone on many levels. I underwent so much pain and many sorrows. I am incredibly grateful for life, and at the same time I know the hardships life sends are far from over.

I live in the present moment more than ever before. I find pleasure in simple things. I feel grace frequently and everywhere around me. In nature, I stop to smell the roses. As the dandelions turn to seed, I pause to pick them, close my eyes, and make a wish before blowing the seeds up into the sky. I relish rainbows, delight in sunsets, and am captivated by every full moon. I see beauty in people, in others' hearts, and also that of my own.

I believe that suffering changed me. I am more compassionate towards my pain and receptive to the tenderness of others. My cancer journey connected me with deep compassion for all and a higher perspective over life's many pain points. I feel compelled to help more. To give a voice to those experiencing a crisis — not just those who have health ailments, like cancer, but in general. I feel compelled to shine a light on the many unseen needs of others.

So, to finally answer my question from above about what is the new normal in life after cancer? I guess that the best way I can sum it all up is to say I'm honestly not sure I've figured it out and am still trying to adjust to my "new normal." Maybe in a few years' time I will have enough experience to write another book about life after cancer; but for now, I can only share what I know so far.

I think, in the end, it really helps to try and stay positive, and to not fret over the days when life gets too tough. Remember, toxic positivity is bad. You might better manage your life and your history with cancer when you're able to look at things from a positive perspective. But that's not always going to be possible.

I also admit my positive attitude can't necessarily stop cancer from growing or prevent it from coming back, but I do know it helps me feel better about life in the present moment and is better for me in general. We all know now that stress is not good to experience long-term, so learning how to cope with surviving cancer and adjusting to life after it is an important measure to work at.

Just remember you don't have to be "happy" all the time. Don't beat yourself up when feelings like guilt, sadness, anger, anxiety, or stress creep in. By this point in the book, you've got an arsenal of tools up your sleeve and tips to help work through surviving life after cancer like a Zen master. Well, at least on most days!

I Hope This Helps

These are some ideas that have helped me deal with uncertainty and fear. Be aware of your many new emotions after treatment, but don't judge them. Practice letting it all go. It's normal for these thoughts to enter your mind, but you don't have to keep them there. Remember to practice observing them and deciding to pick another, and to let the thoughts that plague you float on by and eventually away. However you decide to practice this, letting go of fears about recurrence can free you from wasting valuable energy on needless worry that isn't worth your while -or health.

Live in the present moment. Take it a day at a time rather than thinking about uncertainty around your future or dwelling over difficulties from the past. If you can find a way to feel peaceful inside yourself, even if only for a few minutes a day, try practicing your daily doses of happiness. You can start to recall that sensation of peace whenever life gets too busy, confusing, or downright hard.

That's the best advice I can offer as of now as I am still living in this season. Let's recap what I have learned from my short time in life after treatment as a cancer survivor.

» Finishing treatment is the start of a whole new journey, and for many, not easy to adjust to. It's common to experience a range of emotions and many different feelings after treatment ends.
» Many cancer survivors don't feel the way they expect to feel after treatment ends. You may find you need time to recover not only physically, but emotionally. Life has changed and is not the same as it was before diagnosis. Many people need time to reflect on their cancer experience. With time, most survivors say they find a new, often improved, way of living a new normal.
» Common feelings may include relief, isolation, fear of recurrence, uncertainty, insecurity about the future, frustration with

expectations from family and friends, scanxiety about checkups, worry about late after-effects experienced following cancer treatment, concerns about financial pressures and returning to work, lacking confidence, sadness, confusion, and anger.

Many survivors will discover they need ongoing support after their treatment finishes. Treatment will depend on a person's specific symptoms and situation. It might include therapy, medication, or support groups. Acknowledging and talking about how you're feeling may help you manage your emotions. Communicate often with family, friends, and your doctors if you find yourself struggling and ask for help if you need to.

It's common to experience periods of post-treatment stress and anxiety for months or even years after treatment has ended.

A psychologist recently explained to me that it's common among survivors, following such extreme trauma, to feel like you've had the rug pulled out from underneath you. Questioning your view of the world, and your role in it, happens not only during cancer; many continue to experience this after surviving it. I continue to deeply check in with my core values and beliefs, all while striving to live on purpose and with more meaning following life after treatment. I was assured that this is all perfectly normal and healthy. This was reassuring to hear from a professional psychologist because, by this point in the story, you all know me way too well and could likely question my sanity sometimes, right along with my family members and me!

The bottom line is this: there is little to no sense in trying to go back to life as it was, because doing so could hinder all the progress made after you've changed so much for the better. Falling back into old habits and patterns that were damaging to your health is, obviously, not going to serve you well.

You can't fit a square peg into a round hole, so they say, and you should do your very best to pick up the new and improved pieces of your reshaped life and continue to build upon the better foundation you have since formed, working toward continued momentum and growth. Life as it was may be a far cry from how it should be or from life as you know it today. Chances are, most likely, that you are better off for it.

Lastly, if you are a cancer survivor, try to reflect on this good news and keep in mind that you did it! You are one of the millions alive today who has had cancer and lived to tell your tale. Like most survivors, you and the people around you will adjust to leading a fulfilling life after cancer. A life that is hopefully long but, more importantly, well-lived.

Epilogue

Surviving cancer was anything but easy. Doing it may be the toughest thing I've ever done. Reaching this point is miraculous. Thriving with cancer was maybe the greatest takeaway the entire experience granted me. Learning to live beyond my cancer, growing through it, is remarkable, too, allowing me to become and appreciate a better me. You don't need to reach the light at the end of the tunnel when you can be the light in the midst of the darkness. It's possible to start living your best life today, even during your darkest season.

Learning to live when you feel like you are dying is an extraordinary triumph and one that I'm committed to helping others discover for themselves. I feel it is actually my mission to do this and the very reason why I felt compelled to write this book.

I believe there can be an emotional component behind illness. I believe that, in my case, it was the chronic stress I personally experienced that was the root cause behind my disease. Learning to address this difficulty differently ultimately played a significant role in helping me heal from the inside out.

There are some who might say that my attributing what happened to me being connected to my emotional health is a dangerous assumption to make. They may say that my suggesting my mental and emotional stress had a role in causing the onset of my disease, and that then dealing with it differently had a role in restoring my health, is an unsubstantiated notion. I am not here trying to offer false hope that your belief and thoughts alone can heal such a dangerous disease. What I know for sure is this: it indeed holds tremendous power. It did, at least for me.

I also want to add that I could never have reached this point without the people who, along the way, managed my medical treatment and proposed lifestyle changes that helped restore me back to optimal health. My surgeon, my oncologist, my clean dietary and non-toxic product advisors, and others provided the forms of conventional treatment and complementary alternative therapies that led to my being where I now am today—a far healthier and happier version of my former self.

So much of this journey comes from deep within. There is no one way to optimal health and happiness. It is happiness itself that ultimately is the only way to a life well lived beyond cancer. You must nourish your heart and soul in order to heal your body. That is the key to improved quality of life, the path to living on purpose and with more meaning for what time you have left. Something that is available to us all no matter where we are at in life.

As you reflect on this book, I hope you can now see how you are more than capable of living beyond cancer. I am getting all fired up here, just hoping for you to see how extraordinary you really are. You need to believe in yourself as much as I do. Because I do believe in you. I believe in you wholeheartedly and more than you know.

I know that facing a crisis can be such a lonely and isolating experience. Particularly if your crisis is with cancer. I also want you to know there is an awkward, eclectic, enthusiastic, crazy mom of four cheering for you every step of the way.

I'm over here wishing, praying, hoping, and rooting for you all the way from my home in Southern California. Maybe someday I'll be cheering you on from beaches of Costa Rica as I chase my dreams at Sámara Sueños. Wherever I may be at the time you are reading this, I'm with you right now in spirit.

What you also need to know is that no matter how much I believe in you, none of that really matters -if you don't do so on your own behalf. None of all that we have covered here in this book matters much at all if you haven't learned to believe in your own self. Just like my husband, Will, wasn't able to be with me in the Intensive Care Unit when I arguably needed him most, this is my way of reminding you that this is an inner journey *only* you can make. I'm not going to be there to tell you to get up out of bed—no matter whether that bed is inside of a hospital or your bedroom.

I'm not going to be there when you don't know how you're going to survive another day of cancer treatment or when you show up to start your very first one.

I'm not going to be there to say you'll pass on the steak and potatoes, opting instead for a mouthful of leafy greens and antioxidant-rich fruits and veggies.

I'm not going to be there to clean up your cupboards and detoxify your household and personal care products.

I'm not going to be there on the days when you are feeling most vulnerable, weak, afraid, scared, or hurting.

I'm not going to be there when deeply disappointing interruptions leave you facing an unexpected setback after you were well on your way to wherever it is you had hoped to be.

I'm not going to be there for you when you go to that first post-treatment cancer scan.

I'm not going to be there to hold your hand or help you deal with any or all of your hard stuff.

I'm not going to be there reminding you to channel your inner warrior, to keep on suiting up to battle for life.

You are the only one who is going to be there each and every day that you have left. You'd better believe that your life is well worth fighting for and continue to show up. Doing so may be the hardest and best thing you've ever had to do.

There are going to be a lot of things you are going to have to do, none of which are easy, but many are simple and very doable. When you are just starting off on a journey like this, it can feel incredibly overwhelming. There is no quick fix or way to get where you want to be if you opt for the easy way out.

That's not how it works in life. Some days, the idea of trying to muster through another will feel like more than you have got to give.

It's going to be challenging for sure, but it is possible. Just take it one day at a time, and for the days when that feels too daunting, then take it minute by minute, or moment to moment.

Why keep going when it all seems hopeless? I promise you there is always sunshine on the other side of every storm, and you deserve to at least try to take in the magnificent rainbow. You deserve to live as the best version of yourself and with the greatest quality of life filled with authentic joy and beauty. You deserve to meet the person you were born to be, and maybe this book can be the first step in taking you there.

The time has come where all good things must come to an end, including our time together here.

I went into remission like a firestorm and devoted myself to writing a book with the message that you are in control of your life. You are capable of more than you ever thought possible.

Thank you for accompanying me as I shared the many hard-earned lessons gained from my own journey to health and happiness by detailing everything that I learned along the way.

Each chapter of this book contains a lesson for what I believe either helped me recover from, or contributed to, developing this disease. I identified these primary factors as most instrumental for my own success and felt inspired to share them in my effort to help others facing similar circumstances.

I recently read that the life expectancy for the average American woman is 80 years old. What a blessing it would be to have the great fortune to experience 80 years of life. That said, my story should serve as a stark reminder that this statistic is nothing more than a prediction, not a promise. A long life is what we all may hope for, but it's not a guarantee.

To lead a life well lived for whatever amount of time I may have in it, ideally, a life full of meaning and abundance, has been a long-term goal of mine, reaching back years prior to developing cancer. It was through cancer, however, that I ultimately experienced the pivotal awakening needed to better understand how to actually go about doing so. I put in the hard work required to fully embrace and experience living wholeheartedly.

If you are reading these final words here today, then please know you already have an advantageous set up for continued success. Today offers you the gift of another chance. Every day is an opportunity for you to give back and to become more. When you align your life with your true purpose and passions you will finally achieve all you were created to be.

Thank you for joining me to tell you the tale of how I faced my greatest fear, learned to live courageously—and was fortunate enough to make it through to the other side. I braved the storm, weathered the rain, and am now standing under my own magnificent rainbow, able to share my happy ending.

ABOUT THE AUTHOR

Erin Soto is a Stage 3 cancer survivor, writer, motivational speaker, and wellness advocate. Passionate in her fight against cancer, Erin believes that in order to treat disease, we must treat the whole person—mind, body, and spirit. She inspires countless people to take charge of their health and happiness. She teaches how to navigate life crises by sharing tips and resources using the power of the human spirit and mindset to overcome disaster. Erin lives in Southern California with her husband, William, and their four children.

Hang out with her on Instagram and Facebook
@AuthorErinSoto.

To find out more, follow her No Regrets Blog
and head to **AuthorErinSoto.com.**

Acknowledgments

I have to start by thanking my awesome husband, **William Soto**. From encouraging me to chase this wild idea to offering advice on the cover to keeping the littles out of my hair so I could write, he was as important to this book getting done as I was.

To my four beloved children: **Sienna**, **Cristian**, **Taylor**, and **Liam**: You are my greatest reason for living. You lit up my life the day you came into the world. Here is proof that what was meant to hurt you can always be turned to good. Never give up on chasing your dreams. I hope this story will bring some purpose to our pain and leave us with a lasting legacy we can take pride in together.

To my parents, **Lois** and **Howard Hughes** and **James** and **Irene McDowell,** who are my greatest life advocates: Your unconditional love made me capable of accomplishing far more than I ever could have imagined. Thank you to my Momma for never missing a single appointment throughout my entire cancer journey and for doing so during the insanity of the pandemic. Your insistence on sitting outside of the hospital, waiting in your car during my chemotherapy infusions, mattered more than you realized. Just knowing you were as close as physically possible while with me in spirit carried me through some of the toughest days of treatment. I could never have survived cancer without your unwavering strength and care. I love you.

To **Megan** and **Scott McDowell**, **Kim** and **Keith Wiley**, **Stacy** and **Greg Hansen**, **Allan** and **Jennifer Soto**, **Denise** and **Armando Naylon-Navarette**, **Catalina Soto,** and **Lynne Reed**: Your role in this crazy thing called life that we all share together is such a blessing, and a gift that only family like you could possibly carry. You are all loved beyond measure, as is the rest of our big and beautiful family.

To my real-life heroes. You know exactly who you are, the miracles you have worked, and the lives you have saved: **Jeff David Tracy, MD, Shireena Desai, MD, Jan Beth Schimke, MD,** and **Albert K. Park, MD.**

Thanks to everyone on the publishing team whose expertise and skills helped me so much. Special thanks to **Elaine O'Neill**, the brilliant, ever-so-talented wordsmith who helped fine-tune the messy version of the original manuscript; **Lauren Bittrich**, for polishing it into perfection; **Vanessa Mendozzi**, the greatest cover and interior designer I could ever ask for; **Kristen O'Connell**, whose strategy helped this book find its way to the readers it was intended to serve; and, finally, the entire team at **Verity Audio Productions** for helping me find and use my voice for good.

Thank you to my cancerous colorectal tumor, which presented me with the chance to use my worst life experience as my greatest opportunity to learn and grow with grit and grace. You came crashing in like a wrecking ball obliterating every aspect of life as I knew it, offering up the chance to rebuild a better foundation for a fresh start. While I am happy you are gone for what I hope to be forever, without you I never would have seen the greatest side of so many I know who have since restored my faith in humanity.

Thanks to **Lisa, Matt** and the **Lawkun** family who kept our kids out and about during the early days when we were down in the dumps; **Jed** and **Candice Noll** for being there when the going got tough, a.k.a. my soul sister who never fails to make me laugh so hard I pee my pants IRL. I will never forget our girls' trip to hike the narrows with my cancer-crushing support team of **Paula Dominguez, Pilar Sau Paulo, Leigh Ann Uh,** little **Malory,** and **Taylor,** the nature-basking crew of magical mushies with whom I am grateful to have celebrated my going into remission. To the kind-hearted **Jamie Johnson** and **Elizabeth Sorensen** for packing our many combined kids into one vehicle for carpool rides home from school; **Zeena** and **Azeem Dhalla family** who came to the rescue, arriving at my door immediately following my diagnosis, offering advice and love in more ways than I can ever begin to possibly thank you for; **Arsi** and **Roberto Valenzuela** for keeping my spirits high and friendship close during the season of struggle; **Diana O'Daniel**s, for great company and clean eating inspiration paired with ridiculously fresh produce from farm to our doorstep to celebrate; **Ali Rachel,** for setting me up for this fight feeling loved from an inspirational fellow CRC fighter who knows this dance and sashays across the stage with pure mastery; **Genevieve Rodriguez,** for your amazing photography skills that include this very book cover and years of friendship; **Laurén Earnest,** who made me feel as pretty as I am strong; **Megan** and **Robert Aguilar** for organizing help and meal deliveries early on; **Kim** and **Will Downing**, **Nicole** and **Jason Walsh** who helped our family move from our old house into the apartment including with that ridiculous bedframe you carried up two flights of awkward stairs for the diva cancer patient to rest in; **Heather Brooke** for gifting me with my Crazy, Sexy, Cancer Tips; **Katie Harris** for shipping me the must read When Life Gives You Pears, twice, because the initial package got lost in the mail; **Amy Johansson** for the cozy handmade blanket to snuggle with; **Courtney Nelson** whose vegan cookies and sorbet shipped all the way from Manhattan were the ideal splurge we needed that night to ease our worries. Much gratitude and respect for **Greer Wylder, Si Si Penaloz**a, **Gina Kirschenheiter,** and **Jennifer Heinly** for your generosity in supporting this story in an effort to advocate awareness for and educate others about colorectal cancer. Thank you to the many who offered support to my family and me immediately following my diagnosis. Your donations helped cover initial medical expenses, your thoughtful gifts and tasty meals were thoroughly enjoyed; your caring and prayers mattered so much.

Writing a book is harder than I thought and more rewarding than I ever could have imagined. Although this period of life was filled with many ups and downs, I found the strength to persevere thanks to the many early book backers who believed in my ability to finish this passion project long before the manuscript was complete. This story would not exist without the support of so many who helped to fund the production of this book. Your generosity granted me an opportunity to work with the very best in the business. I'm eternally grateful to you all for playing your part in getting here: **Karen Hagen, Diane** and **Richard Wolak, Lauren Roll, Rick Wesslund, Kelly Erickson, Nicole** and **Jason Murray, Erica** and **Jim Hume, Esmeralda** and **César Loya, Kati McIlroy, Gina Urquizu, Denyce Griffin, Jennifer Kearney, Penny** and **Jeff Williams, Allison Cabral, Jessica Elliot, Jill Dougherty, Steve Carlton, Mike Blanchard, Jackie Bartel, Stephanie** and **Jim Abbot, Eileen McEuen, Jennifer Blose**, the one and only **Janine** (J-9), **Leslie Waggoner, Christina Darnell, Brooks Keith, Norman** and **Ann Harck, Peggy Levien, Steve Wilson, Lize Biersch, Tricia** and **Michael Schanna, Stephanie Hunt, Gina Stassi, Jodey Dugan, Swan Nguyen, Alan Avery, Jeff Schwartzman, Tim va Ee, Ashley Mendell, Bob Mantey, Michelle Swint, Joseph Fordonski, Ken Silverman, Kristen Silka** and **Sandra Bertola**.

NOTES

PART I: WHEN THE STUDENT IS READY, THE TEACHER ARRIVES

1. Simon, Stacy. "Colorectal Cancer Rates Rise in Younger Adults." *American Cancer Society*, March 05, 2020. https://www.cancer.org/latest-news/colorectal-cancer-rates-rise-in-younger-adults.html.
2. Underferth, Danielle. "What Young Adults Need to Know About Colorectal Cancer." *The University of Texas MD Anderson Cancer Center*, October 27, 2020. www.mdanderson.org/cancerwise/why-are-more-young-adults-getting-colorectal-cancer-what-to-know.h00-159385890.html.
3. PDQ® Adult Treatment Editorial Board. "PDQ Colon Cancer Treatment." Bethesda, MD: National Cancer Institute. Updated December 20, 2021. https://www.cancer.gov/types/colorectal/patient/colon-treatment-pdq. [PMID: 26389319].
4. "Cancer Facts & Figures 2021." *American Cancer Society*, March 05, 2021. https://www.cancer.org/content/dam/cancer-org/research/cancer-facts-and-statistics/annual-cancer-facts-and-figures/2021/cancer-facts-and-figures-2021.pdf
5. *"Cancer Statistics." National Cancer Institute, September 25, 2020. https://www.cancer.gov/about-cancer/understanding/statistics*

PART II: HOW TO HEAL THE MIND

1. "Nothing Is Solid & Everything Is Energy, According to New Research." *Power of Positivity*, July 16, 2016. https://www.powerofpositivity.com/physicists-prove-that-nothing-is-solid/
2. Tseng, J., Poppenk, J. "Brain meta-state transitions demarcate thoughts across task contexts exposing the mental noise of trait neuroticism." *Nat Commun* 11, 3480 (2020). https://doi.org/10.1038/s41467-020-17255-9

PART III: HOW TO HEAL THE BODY

1. "Nutrition and Healthy Eating."*Mayo Clinic*, October 30, 2019. https://www.mayoclinic.org/healthy-lifestyle/nutrition-and-healthy-eating/in-depth/how-plant-based-food-helps-fight-cancer/art-20457590
2. Tantamango-Bartley, Yessenia and Jaceldo-Siegl, Karen and Fan, Jing and Fraser, Gary. *"Vegetarian diets and the incidence of cancer in a low-risk population."* National Library of Medicine, November 20, 2012. https://pubmed.ncbi.nlm.nih.gov/23169929/
3. Key, Timothy and Appleby, Paul and Spencer, Elizabeth and Travis, Ruth and Roddam, Andrew and Allen, Naomi. "Cancer Incidence in Vegetarians: Results from the European Prospective Investigation into Cancer and Nutrition (EPIC-Oxford)." *National Library of Medicine*, March 11, 2009. https://pubmed.ncbi.nlm.nih.gov/19279082/.
4. Freston, Kathy. "A Vegan Diet (Hugely) Helpful Against Cancer." *Huff Post*, December 12, 2012. https://www.huffpost.com/entry/vegan-diet-cancer_b_2250052
5. Greger, Michael M.D. FACLM. "The Answer to the Pritikin Puzzle." *NutritionFacts.org*. September 27, 2012. https://nutritionfacts.org/video/the-answer-to-the-pritikin-puzzle/.
6. Barnard, James and Gonzalez, Jenny, and Liva, Maud and Ngo, Tung. "Effects of a low-fat, high-fiber diet and exercise program on breast cancer risk factors in vivo and tumor cell growth and apoptosis in vitro." *National Library of Medicine*, 2006. https://pubmed.ncbi.nlm.nih.gov/16965238/.
7. Greger, Michael M.D. FACLM. "Slowing the Growth of Cancer." August 20, 2007. https://nutritionfacts.org/video/slowing-the-growth-of-cancer-3/
8. Greger, Michael M.D. FACLM. "Do Vegetarians Get Enough Protein?" *NutritionFacts.org*. June 06, 2014. https://nutritionfacts.org/video/do-vegetarians-get-enough-protein/

Books

1. Turner, Kelly, A. Ph.D. *Radical Remission.* New York, NY: HarperOne, 2015.
2. Dyer, Wayne W. *There's a Spiritual Solution to Every Problem.* New York, NY: HarperCollins, 2003.
3. Dyer, Wayne W. *There's a Spiritual Solution to Every Problem.* New York, NY: Harper, 2001.
4. Chopra, Deepak. *Quantum Healing (Revised and Updated): Exploring the Frontiers of Mind/Body Medicine.* New York, NY: Bantam, 2015.
5. Buchheit, Carl Ph.D. and Schamber, Ellie Ph.D. *Transformational NLP: A New Psychology.* Oregon: White Cloud Press, 2017.
6. Carr, Kris. *Crazy Sexy Cancer Tips.* Charleston, SC: Skirt! Books, An Imprint of Globe Pequot Press, 2007.
7. Carr, Kris and Sarno, Chad. *Crazy Sexy Kitchen.* Charleston, SC: Skirt! Books, An Imprint of Globe Pequot Press, 2011.
8. Werner-Gray, Liana. *The Earth Diet.* Carlsbad, CA: Hay House Inc., 2014.
9. Werner-Gray, Liana. *Cancer-Free With Food.* Carlsbad, CA: Hay House Inc., 2019.
10. Schucman, Helen. *A Course in Miracles.* Novato, CA: Foundation for Inner Peace; 3rd edition, 2007.
11. Moorjani, Anita. *Dying to Be Me: My Journey from Cancer, to Near Death, to True Healing.* Carlsbad, CA: Hayhouse, 2012.

WEBSITES

- Visit my website for more tips and resources on wholehearted wellness, recipes, shop Mother Fighter merchandise for cancer care packages and gifts or read the latest from my blog. A portion of every purchase helps to donate cancer care packages to patients: https://www.authorerinsoto.com/
- If you are interested in supporting Sámara Sueños, please visit: https://www.samarasuenos.org/
- The Think Dirty® app is the easiest way to learn ingredients in your beauty, personal care, and household products. Just scan the product barcode, and Think Dirty will give you easy-to-understand info on the product, its ingredients, and shop cleaner options: https://thinkdirtyapp.com/
- Calm is an excellent app to try for guided meditation, sleep and relaxation: https://www.calm.com/
- Visit the American Institute of Stress to assess your score with Holmes-Rahe Stress Inventory Test: https://www.stress.org/holmes-rahe-stress-inventory
- Transformational Neuro-Linguistic Programming (NLP) is a groundbreaking synthesis of psychology and study of the structure of human experience: https://www.nlpmarin.com/
- *The Game Changers* is a popular documentary featuring visionary scientists and top athletes on a quest to find the optimal diet for human performance and health: https://www.netflix.com/title/81157840
- One of my most favorite kundalini mantras to chant. My family all loves Jai-Jagdeesh's hypnotic Aad Guray Nameh which calms us all: https://open.spotify.com/track/2HnyViFe3CzgZzrQlWCRA1

CPSIA information can be obtained
at www.ICGtesting.com
Printed in the USA
FSHW020121250122
87879FS